Cholesterol and Atherosclerosis

DIAGNOSIS AND TREATMENT

Cholesterol and Atherosclerosis

DIAGNOSIS AND TREATMENT

SCOTT M. GRUNDY, MD, PhD

Director, Center for Human Nutrition
Chairman, Department of Clinical Nutrition
Professor of Internal Medicine and Biochemistry
The University of Texas
Southwestern Medical Center
Dallas, Texas

WITH ORIGINAL ILLUSTRATIONS BY LAURA PARDI DUPREY

J.B. Lippincott Company • Philadelphia
Gower Medical Publishing • New York • London

Distributed in USA and Canada by:
J.B. Lippincott Company
East Washington Square
Philadelphia, PA 19105 USA

Distributed in UK and Continental Europe by:
Harper & Row Ltd
Middlesex House
34-42 Cleveland Street
London W1P 5FB UK

Distributed in Australia and New Zealand by:
Harper & Row (Australia) Pty Ltd
P.O. Box 226
Artarmon, NSW 2064, Australia

Distributed in Southeast Asia, Hong Kong, India, and Pakistan by:
Harper & Row Publishers (Asia) Pte Ltd
37 Jalan Pemimpin 02-01
Singapore 2057

Distributed in Japan by:
Igaku Shoin Ltd
Tokyo International
P.O. Box 5063
Tokyo, Japan

ISBN 0-397-44674-8

10 9 8 7 6 5 4 3 2 1

Editor: William J. Gabello

Illustrator: Laura Pardi Duprey

Designers: Thomas Tedesco, Kathryn Greenslade

Printed and bound in Singapore by
Imago Productions (FE) PTE Ltd.

Library of Congress Cataloging-in-Publication Data

Grundy, Scott M.
    Cholesterol and atherosclerosis : diagnosis and treatment / Scott M. Grundy.
      p. cm.
    Includes bibliographical references.
    ISBN 0-397-44674-8
    1. Hypercholesteremia. 2. Hyperlipidemia. 3. Atherosclerosis—Etiology. 4. Coronary heart disease—Etiology. I. Title.
    [DNLM: 1. Arteriosclerosis—metabolism. 2. Cholesterol—metabolism. 3. Hyperlipidemia—diet therapy. 4. Hyperlipidemia—drug therapy. WG 550 G547c]
RC632.H83G78 1990
616.1'36071—dc20
DNLM/DLC
for Library of Congress
        89-71405

Figure Credits

Fig. 1.4 Modified from Grundy SM: Cholesterol metabolism in man. *West J Med* 128:13–25, 1978.

Fig. 1.18 Based on description by Havel RJ: Origin, metabolic fate, and metabolic function of plasma lipoproteins, in Steinberg D, Olefsky JM (eds): *Hypercholesterolemia and Atherosclerosis: Pathogenesis and Prevention.* Churchill Livingstone, New York, 1987, pp 117–141.

Figs. 1.23, 1.24 Modified from Brown MS, Goldstein JL (1986), see Further Readings, p II.

Fig. 1.29 Modified from Grundy SM, Vega GL (1987), see Further Readings, p V.

Figs. 1.35, 1.36 Modified from Grundy SM (1983), see Further Readings, p II.

Fig. 1.38 Adapted from Keys A (1970), see Further Readings, p II.

Fig. 1.40 Modified from Martin MJ, Hulley SB, Browner WS, et al (1986), see Further Readings, p III.

Fig. 1.41 Adapted from Lipid Research Clinics Program. The Lipid Research Clinics Coronary Primary Prevention Trial results. I and II (1984), see Further Readings, p V. (Kindly made available by Dr. Basil M. Rifkind)

Fig. 1.44 Modified from Malenka DJ, Baron JA: Cholesterol and coronary heart disease: the importance of patient-specific attributable risk. *Arch Intern Med* 148:2247–2252, 1988.

Fig. 1.45 Modified from Anderson KM, Castelli WP, Levy DL: Cholesterol and mortality: 30 years of follow-up from the Framingham Study. *JAMA* 257:2176–2180, 1987.

Figs. 1.46, 1.47, 1.48, 1.50, 1.51 Adapted from the data in several publications from the Framingham Heart Study.

Fig. 1.53 Modified from Grundy SM: Can modification of risk factors reduce coronary heart disease?, in Rahimtoola SH (ed): *Controversies in Coronary Artery Disease*; and Brest AN (ed): *Cardiovascular Clinics*, FA Davis, Philadelphia, 1982, pp 283–296.

Fig. 2.4 Adapted from The Lipid Research Clinics Population Studies Data Book. Vol 1, The Prevalence Study. NIH Publication No. 79-1527. Bethesda, MD, July 1979.

Fig. 2.24 Modified from Brown MS, Goldstein JL (1986), see Further Readings, p II.

Fig. 3.10 Adapted from Keys A (1970), see Further Readings, p II.

Figs. 4.11, 4.13, 4.14 Modified from Rifkind BM, Gordon DJ: Effects of resins on clinical cardiovascular endpoints, in Fears R, Prous JR (eds): *Pharmacological Control of Hyperlipidemia.* Science Publishers, Barcelona, 1986, pp 21–34. (Data derived from Lipid Research Clinics Study; see credit for Fig. 1.41).

Fig. 4.20 Modified from Tobert JA: New developments in lipid-lowering therapy: the role of inhibitors of hydroxymethyl-glutaryl-coenzyme A reductase. *Circulation* 76:534–538, 1987.

Fig. 4.21 Modified from Grundy SM: HMG CoA reductase inhibitors for treatment of hypercholesterolemia. *N Engl J Med* 319:24–33, 1988.

Fig. 4.33 Modified from Frick MH, et al (1987), see Further Readings, p V.

Preface

High serum cholesterol is a major cause of coronary atherosclerosis leading to coronary heart disease (CHD). Although evidence to support a cholesterol–atherosclerosis link has been accumulating for the past century, the past three decades have witnessed a geometrical growth in information about this link. The evidence comes from many sources. It comes from studies in laboratory animals, epidemiologic surveys, studies of genetic disorders of cholesterol metabolism, clinical investigations, and large-scale clinical trials. The evidence that high cholesterol levels are a cause of CHD is widely accepted as proof by most investigators in the field. There is also a growing consensus that therapeutic lowering of serum cholesterol levels will reduce the risk for CHD.

One of the major discoveries in the field of lipid research is that cholesterol is transported in the bloodstream by particles called lipoproteins. Three types of lipoproteins have emerged as playing key roles in atherogenesis. The major cholesterol-carrying lipoprotein is low-density lipoprotein (LDL). High serum levels of LDL promote the development of atherosclerosis. In 1985, Drs. Joseph Goldstein and Michael Brown, of The University of Texas Southwestern Medical Center at Dallas, were awarded the Nobel Prize in Medicine for the discovery of LDL receptors. These proteins, located on the surface of liver cells, remove LDL from the circulation and in this way regulate serum concentrations of LDL; they are thus important determinants of the atherosclerotic process. The research of Drs. Goldstein and Brown has helped bring cholesterol research into the molecular age, and has provided a rational foundation for the management of high serum cholesterol levels.

Another lipoprotein intimately related to atherogenesis is high-density lipoprotein (HDL). In contrast to LDL, high levels of HDL may actually protect against the development of atherosclerosis. The way in which a high HDL level protects against CHD has not yet been determined. Some investigators believe that HDL particles actually remove excess cholesterol from coronary arteries and thereby retard atherogenesis. Other workers are of the opinion that a low HDL level merely reflects an excess of other, atherogenic lipoproteins, notably, very low-density lipoproteins (VLDL), which are the major carriers of triglycerides in the circulation. Recent data of several types suggest that high levels of VLDL impart an increased risk for CHD.

Strong evidence has existed for many years that high serum levels of total cholesterol and LDL-cholesterol promote the development of atherosclerosis. Until recently, however, it has been questionable whether therapeutic modification of lipoproteins actually will reduce the risk for CHD. This question has largely been answered in the affirmative by two large clinical trials: the Lipid Research Clinics Coronary Primary Prevention Trial, which used cholestyramine as a cholesterol-lowering drug, and the Helsinki Heart Study, which employed gemfibrozil. In both trials, individuals receiving the respective drugs exhibited reduced rates of CHD in comparison with those receiving placebo. On the basis of previous support for a cholesterol–atherosclerosis link and the results of these and other clinical trials, the National Institutes of Health sponsored a National Cholesterol Education Program. The purpose of this program is to increase awareness among health professionals and the general public of the dangers of a high serum cholesterol, and to provide information on how best to manage high cholesterol levels. The program urges all adults over age 20 to have their blood cholesterol checked by their physician and, if the level is high, to seek appropriate treatment.

Abundant evidence indicates that the typical American diet is the primary cause of "mass hypercholesterolemia" in the United States; the same holds for other "high-risk" populations. Therefore, the first line of therapy for elevated serum cholesterol is dietary modification. Three dietary factors raise the serum cholesterol concentration: saturated fatty acids, cholesterol, and excess total calories resulting in obesity. If high-risk populations will gradually alter their eating habits, serum cholesterol levels should decline, resulting in an overall decrease in coronary risk. However, individuals found to have high cholesterol levels, particularly elevations of the LDL-cholesterol fraction, should undergo dietary modification under physician supervision in an effort to reduce their LDL levels to acceptable values. Some individuals may find it easier to modify their diets with the assistance of a registered dietitian. Dietary modification alone should be adequate to manage the majority of people with elevated serum cholesterol.

Even though most people with high serum cholesterol should respond adequately to dietary therapy, substantial numbers of people have genetic forms of dyslipidemia, which make them candidates for drug therapy. Various drugs are now available for treatment of high serum lipids. Recently, new drugs have been introduced that are extremely potent for lowering serum cholesterol and apparently carry no serious side effects. Cholesterol-lowering drugs must be used judiciously, but in people with genetic disorders of lipid metabolism, drugs may act to extend life.

The cholesterol–atherosclerosis connection is simple in concept but complex in reality. The connection is mediated through a complicated system of lipoproteins and their interactions within the arterial wall. Further, high serum cholesterol is only one of several other major risk factors for CHD. The purpose of this book is to present the complex biochemical and physiologic pathways of lipoproteins in a clear and graphic manner. Its excellent illustrations show how abnormalities in lipoprotein metabolism are responsible for development of various dyslipidemias. They also indicate the mechanisms whereby therapeutic diets and drugs modify lipoprotein metabolism. This book should be a useful adjunct to physicians and other health professionals in their management of patients with dyslipidemia. People who have inherited high blood cholesterol or triglyceride levels may find the book valuable for understanding the metabolic basis of their disorder. The book also contains useful tips on the selection of foods to lower the blood cholesterol.

S.M.G.

Unit One

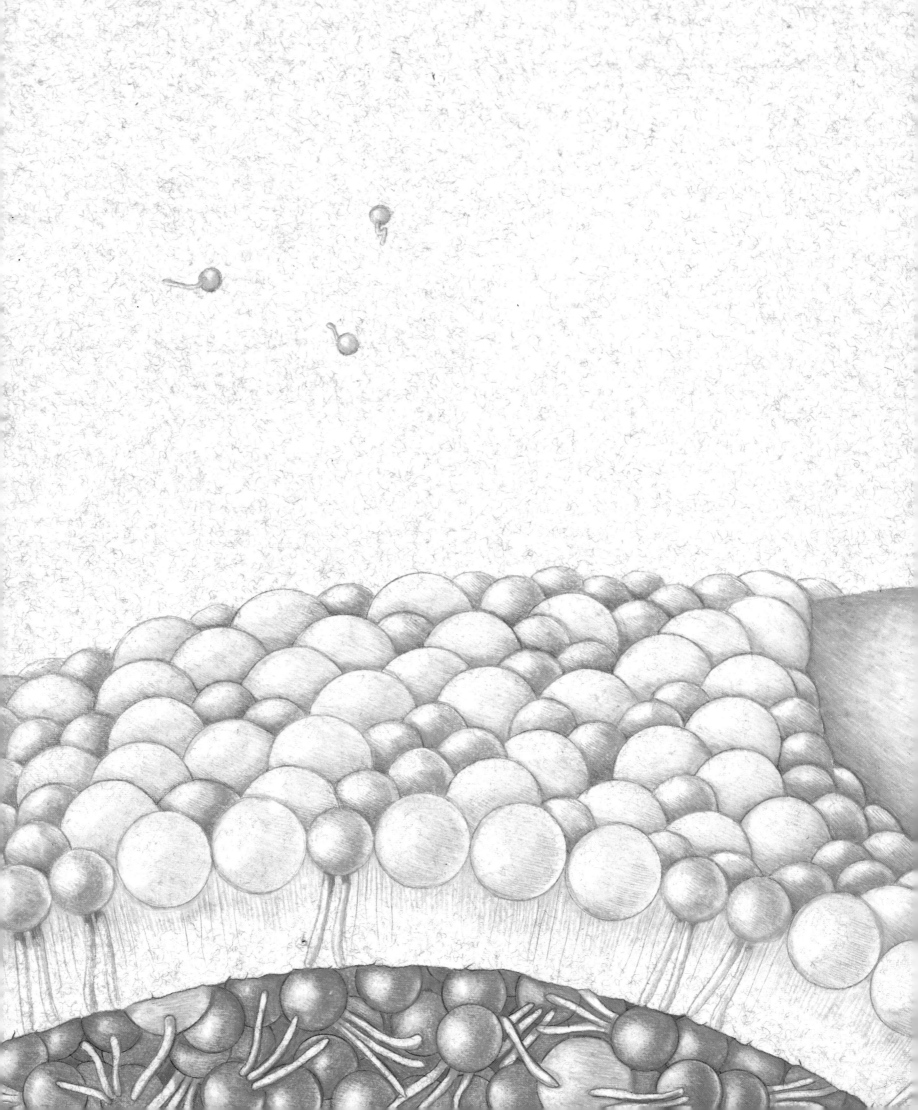

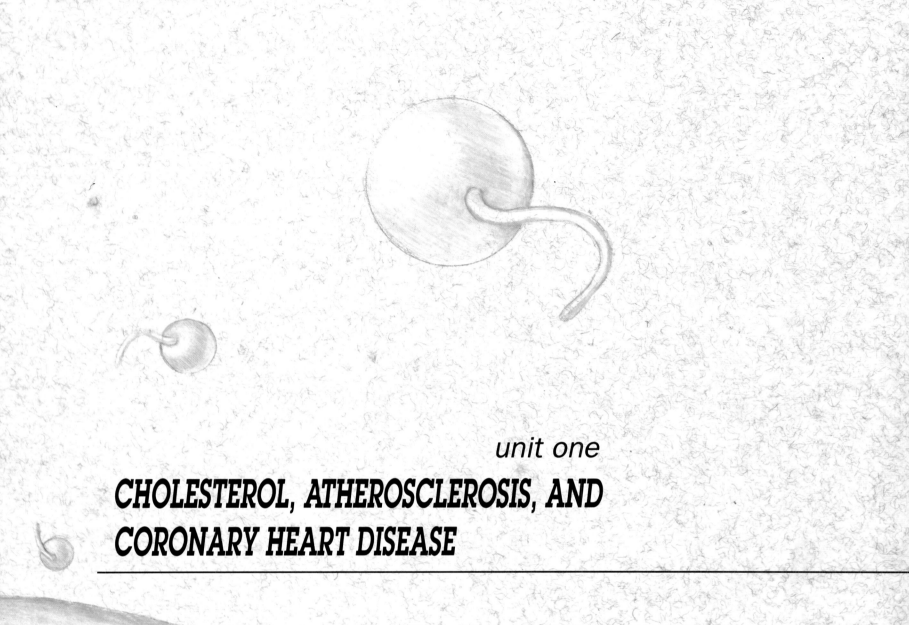

unit one

CHOLESTEROL, ATHEROSCLEROSIS, AND
CORONARY HEART DISEASE

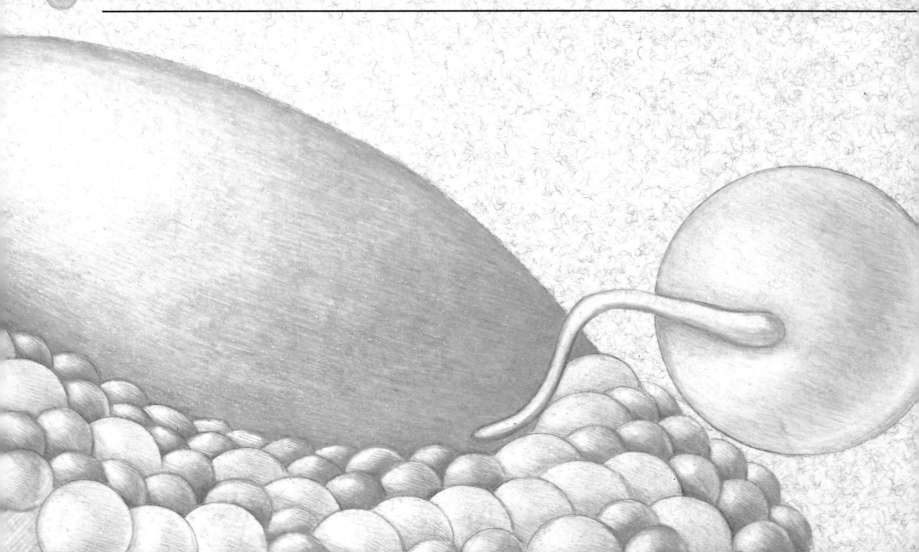

A high blood (serum) cholesterol level is a major risk factor for coronary heart disease (CHD). The reason for this is that excess cholesterol in the circulation promotes the development of coronary atherosclerosis, the most common condition underlying CHD. A link between cholesterol and CHD has been firmly established through many lines of evidence. Recently, it has been documented that therapeutic lowering of serum cholesterol delays or prevents the occurrence of CHD. These findings justify efforts to control high cholesterol levels through detection and treatment of patients with definitely elevated cholesterol and through modification of lifestyles of the general public. Effective treatment of high serum cholesterol in its many forms requires a good grasp by physicians of the underlying metabolism of cholesterol and the pathophysiology of its link to CHD. This unit provides the necessary background for understanding the causes of high serum cholesterol and the clinical approaches to its management.

CHOLESTEROL METABOLISM

STRUCTURE OF CHOLESTEROL AND RELATED LIPIDS

Cholesterol is an insoluble lipid containing a steroid-ring nucleus. It has one hydroxy group and one double-bond in the steroid nucleus, together with a side chain of eight carbon atoms (Fig. 1.1). Cholesterol is structurally different from the other major lipids of the body, triglycerides and phospholipids, both of which have fatty acids as their major constituent. Moreover, depending on the number of double-bonds, the fatty acids may be saturated (no double-bonds), monounsaturated (one double-bond), or polyunsaturated (two or more double-bonds).

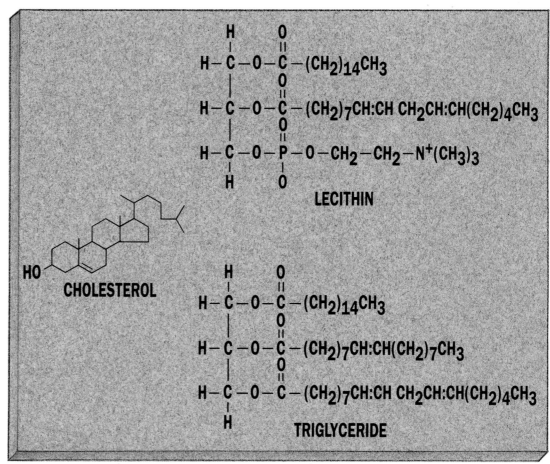

Fig. 1.1 Structure of cholesterol in comparison with structures of other major lipids, lecithin and triglyceride.

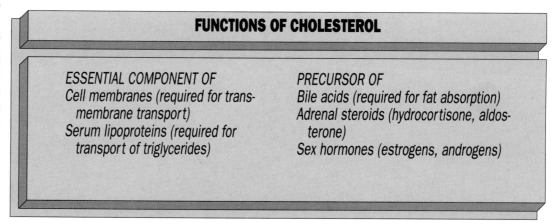

Fig. 1.2 Functions of cholesterol.

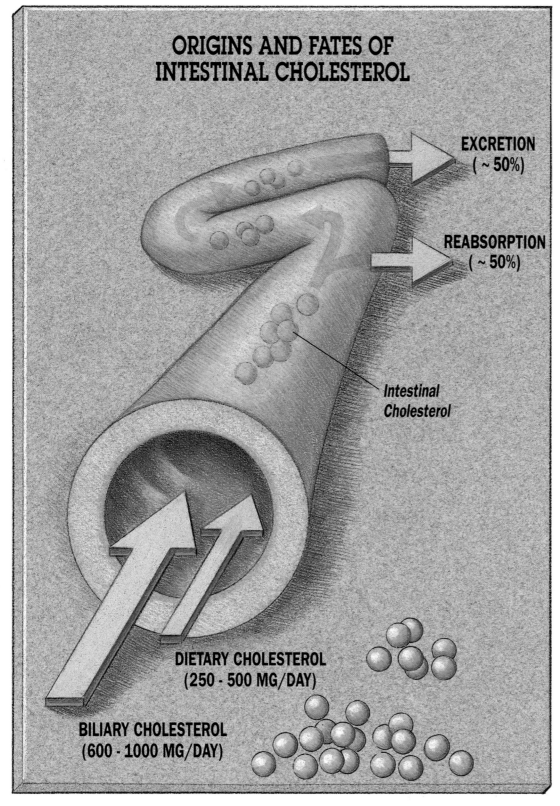

FUNCTIONS OF CHOLESTEROL

Cholesterol has several vital functions in the body (Fig. 1.2). It is an essential component of most cell membranes of the body, providing stability and allowing for transmembrane transport. Cholesterol is especially necessary as a membrane constituent in the central nervous system where it is present in abundance. It also plays an important role in the transport of triglycerides in the serum by being an essential component of serum lipoproteins (see discussion below). It is the precursor of bile acids, which are synthesized in the liver and participate in the absorption of fat in the intestine. Finally, cholesterol is the precursor of the adrenal steroids (hydrocortisone and aldosterone) and sex hormones (estrogens and androgens). Thus, without adequate quantities of cholesterol in the body, survival would not be possible.

ORIGINS AND FATES OF INTESTINAL CHOLESTEROL

Cholesterol entering the intestine originates from either the bile or the diet (Fig. 1.3). In adults, input of biliary cholesterol ranges from 600 to 1000 mg per day, whereas dietary intake of cholesterol varies between 250 and 500 mg per day. All dietary cholesterol is of animal origin. Plants do not produce cholesterol; instead, the cell membranes of plants contain another sterol, sitosterol, of which the average diet contains 100 to 200 mg per day. Cholesterol entering the intestine can have two fates: normally, about 50% is absorbed, and the remainder is excreted in stools.

Fig. 1.3 Origins and fates of intestinal cholesterol.

Fig. 1.4 Mechanism of cholesterol absorption.

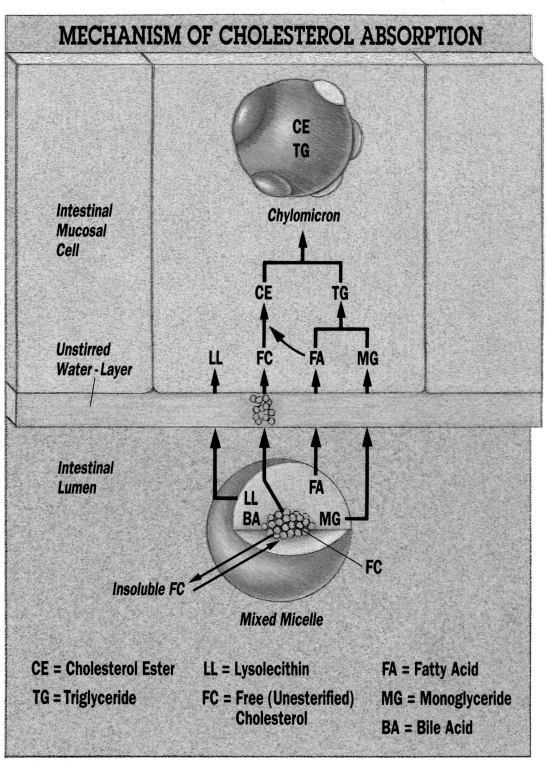

MECHANISM OF CHOLESTEROL ABSORPTION

Chylomicron

Intestinal Mucosal Cell

Unstirred Water-Layer

Intestinal Lumen

Insoluble FC

Mixed Micelle

CE = Cholesterol Ester

TG = Triglyceride

LL = Lysolecithin

FC = Free (Unesterified) Cholesterol

FA = Fatty Acid

MG = Monoglyceride

BA = Bile Acid

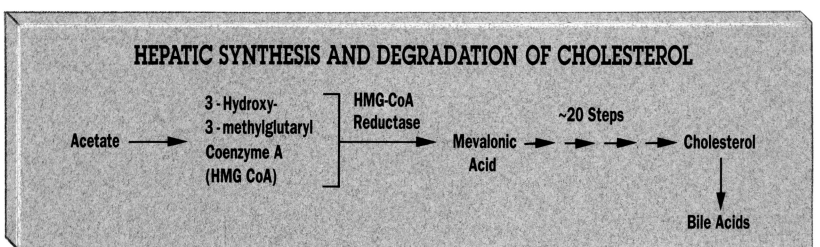

HEPATIC SYNTHESIS AND DEGRADATION OF CHOLESTEROL

Acetate → 3-Hydroxy-3-methylglutaryl Coenzyme A (HMG CoA) → HMG-CoA Reductase → Mevalonic Acid → ~20 Steps → Cholesterol → Bile Acids

Fig. 1.5 Hepatic synthesis and degradation of cholesterol.

1.4 Cholesterol, Atherosclerosis, and Coronary Heart Disease

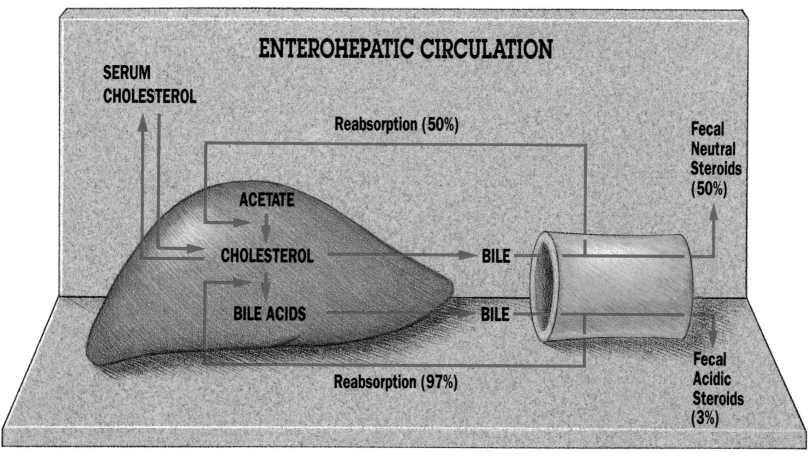

Fig. 1.6 Enterohepatic circulation: continuous cycling of cholesterol and bile acids between the intestine and the liver.

MECHANISMS OF CHOLESTEROL ABSORPTION

Since cholesterol is so highly insoluble in aqueous systems, special mechanisms are required for its absorption by the intestine (Fig. 1.4). Within the intestinal lumen, cholesterol is solubilized into mixed micelles containing fatty acids and monoglycerides (derived from hydrolysis of dietary triglycerides), lecithin, lysolecithin, and bile acids. All of these lipids act like detergents to hold cholesterol in solution and bring it into proximity to the mucosal cell. Cholesterol must then traverse a thin, unstirred water-layer by monomolecular diffusion to enter the outer membrane of intestinal mucosal cells. All of the polar lipids in the lumen participate in the solubilization of cholesterol, but bile acids are absolutely necessary; without them, cholesterol cannot be absorbed. When the polar lipids themselves are absorbed, cholesterol falls out of solution and cannot be absorbed; this explains why only about 50% of cholesterol in the intestinal lumen is actually absorbed.

HEPATIC SYNTHESIS AND DEGRADATION OF CHOLESTEROL

The liver is a major site of cholesterol synthesis in the body, although choles- terol also is produced in many other organs and tissues. All cholesterol is derived ultimately from acetate (Fig. 1.5). Three molecules of the latter are condensed to produce 3-hydroxy-3-methylglutaryl coenzyme A (HMG CoA), which in turn is converted to mevalonic acid through the action of the enzyme HMG-CoA reductase. This reaction is the rate-limiting step in the biosynthesis of cholesterol. Through a series of condensations and rearrangements, mevalonic acid is transformed into cholesterol. In the liver, cholesterol is partially degraded into the primary bile acids, cholic acid and chenodeoxycholic acid. The bile acids assist in removal of cholesterol from the body by contributing to its solubilization in bile, the major route of cholesterol excretion.

ENTEROHEPATIC CIRCULATION

Cholesterol and bile acids cycle continuously between the intestine and the liver in a process known as the enterohepatic circulation (Fig. 1.6). In the liver, cholesterol synthesized from acetate can have three fates: It can (1) enter the serum, (2) be converted into bile acids, or (3) be secreted into the bile and hence into the intestine. When cholesterol enters the intestine, approximately 50% is reabsorbed and returns to the liver; the remainder is excreted into stools as fecal neutral steroids. The amount of cholesterol returning to the liver controls, by feedback regulation, the amount of new cholesterol synthesized. A high return of cholesterol to the liver suppresses the activity of HMG-CoA reductase and thereby inhibits cholesterol synthesis. If less cholesterol returns to the liver, the activity of HMG-CoA reductase is increased, and more cholesterol is synthesized. This feedback regulation thus functions to maintain an optimal amount of cholesterol in liver cells.

The bile acids, likewise, have an enterohepatic circulation. They too are secreted into bile and hence into the intestine. In the bile, they help solubilize biliary cholesterol; in the intestine, they promote absorption of both fat and cholesterol. Normally, about 97% to 98% of bile acids is reabsorbed in the lower intestine, and only about 3% is excreted in stools as fecal acidic steroids. The bile acids are reabsorbed into the portal circulation and are largely extracted in their first pass through the liver. In the liver, the bile acids regulate their own synthesis rate by feedback regulation. In most adults, about 300 to 500 mg of cholesterol are converted into bile acids each day. The bile acids are resecreted into bile to complete the enterohepatic circulation. On average,

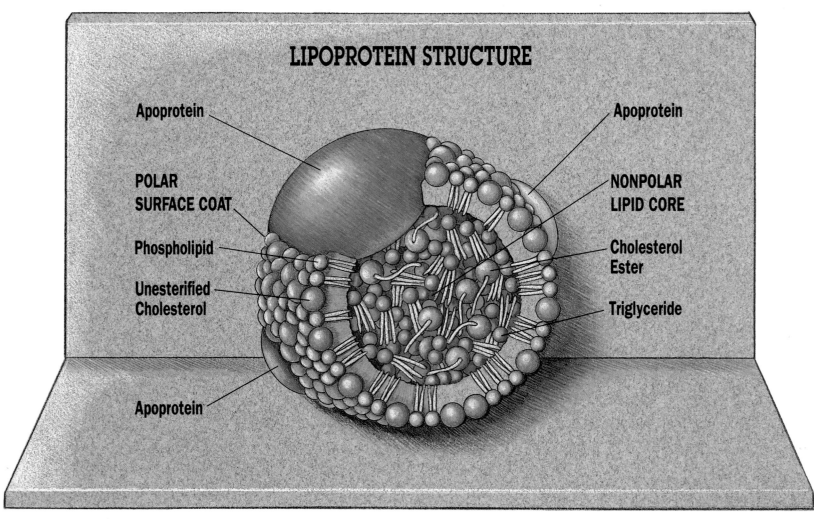

LIPOPROTEIN STRUCTURE

Apoprotein

Apoprotein

POLAR SURFACE COAT

NONPOLAR LIPID CORE

Phospholipid

Cholesterol Ester

Unesterified Cholesterol

Triglyceride

Apoprotein

Fig. 1.7 Basic structure of lipoproteins.

bile acids recycle in the enterohepatic circulation about six times per day — twice with each meal.

CHOLESTEROL TRANSPORT

Since cholesterol is so highly insoluble in aqueous solutions, it cannot circulate freely in plasma. Instead, it must be transported in molecular complexes called *lipoproteins*. These particles contain both lipids and proteins, the latter named *apolipoproteins* (apoproteins). Several classes of lipoproteins are involved in cholesterol transport, and in some cases, these same lipoproteins carry triglycerides. Indeed, from the point of view of energy metabolism, the transport of triglycerides may be the

more important function. In the sections that follow, the structure and function of the various lipoproteins involved in transport of cholesterol and triglycerides are examined.

LIPOPROTEIN STRUCTURE

The basic structures of all lipoproteins are similar; they all contain a core of neutral lipids consisting of cholesterol esters and triglycerides, a surface coat of more polar lipids — unesterified cholesterol and phospholipids — and apoproteins (Fig. 1.7). The surface coat, whose lipids provide a covering structure that resembles the typical plasma membrane of cells, serves as an interface between the aqueous

plasma and the inner nonpolar lipid core. This polar surface thus makes possible the transport of the highly insoluble cholesterol esters and triglycerides in plasma. The apoproteins of the surface coat serve several important functions:

1. They are required for the synthesis and secretion of specific lipoproteins.
2. They act to stabilize the surface coat and hence the whole lipoprotein particle.
3. They are cofactors in the activation of enzymes that modify the lipoproteins.
4. They can interact with specific cell-surface receptors that remove lipoproteins from the circulation.

CLASSIFICATION OF LIPOPROTEINS

LIPOPROTEIN	DENSITY (g/ml)	SOURCES
Chylomicrons	~0.98	Intestine
Very low - density lipoproteins (VLDL) (prebetalipoproteins)	~1.006	Liver
Intermediate - density lipoproteins (IDL)	1.006 – 1.019	Catabolism of VLDL
Low - density lipoproteins (LDL) (betalipoproteins)	1.019 – 1.063	Catabolism of IDL
High - density lipoproteins (HDL) (alphalipoproteins)	1.063 – 1.21	Liver, intestine, other

Fig. 1.8 Classification of lipoproteins.

APOPROTEIN B'S

APOPROTEIN	MOLECULAR WEIGHT (daltons)	SOURCES	LIPOPROTEINS
B - 48	264,000	Intestine	Chylomicrons
B - 100	550,000	Liver	VLDL, IDL, LDL

Fig. 1.9 Apoprotein B's.

APOPROTEIN A'S

APOPROTEIN	MOLECULAR WEIGHT (daltons)	SOURCES	LIPOPROTEINS
A - I	28,000	Intestine, liver	HDL, chylomicrons
A - II	17,000	Intestine, liver	HDL, chylomicrons
A - IV	46,000	Intestine	HDL, chylomicrons

Fig. 1.10 Apoprotein A's.

The apoproteins vary from one lipoprotein to another, and to a large extent, they direct the function of the whole lipoprotein.

LIPOPROTEIN CLASSES

The five major classes of lipoproteins are named either by their density or by their electrophoretic mobility (Fig. 1.8). *Chylomicrons* are triglyceride-rich lipoproteins synthesized by the intestine; they have a density (d) of approximately 0.98 g/ml. *Very low-density lipoproteins* (VLDL) (d < 1.006 g/ml) are triglyceride-rich lipoproteins made by the liver; on electrophoresis they show prebeta mobility. *Intermediate-density lipoproteins* (IDL) (d = 1.006–1.019 g/ml) are produced by the catabolism of VLDL. *Low-density lipoproteins* (LDL) (d = 1.019–1.063 g/ml), which are derived by catabolism of IDL, are the major cholesterol-carrying lipoproteins of serum; they have beta mobility on electrophoresis. Finally, *high-density lipoproteins* (HDL) (d = 1.063–1.21 g/ml), which have alpha mobility, comprise several components derived from various sources—the liver, intestine, other lipoproteins, and other tissue.

APOPROTEINS

Of the four major categories of apoproteins, those with the highest molecular weights are the apoprotein (apo) B's (Fig. 1.9). Apo B-48, produced by the intestine, is present on chylomicrons, whereas apo B-100, which is synthesized by the liver, is a constituent of the surface coat of VLDL, IDL, and LDL. The apo A's, on the other hand, are made by both liver and intestine and are found on chylomicrons and HDL (Fig. 1.10). The

APOPROTEIN C'S

APOPROTEIN	MOLECULAR WEIGHT (daltons)	SOURCES	LIPOPROTEINS
C-I	5,800	Liver	Chylomicrons, VLDL, IDL, HDL
C-II	9,100	Liver	Chylomicrons, VLDL, IDL, HDL
C-III	8,750	Liver	Chylomicrons, VLDL, IDL, HDL

Fig. 1.11 Apoprotein C's.

APOPROTEIN E'S

APOPROTEIN	MOLECULAR WEIGHT (daltons)	POSITION 112	POSITION 158	SOURCES	LIPOPROTEINS
E-2	35,000	Cys	Cys	Liver, peripheral tissues	Chylomicrons, VLDL IDL, HDL
E-3	35,000	Cys	Arg	Liver, peripheral tissues	Chylomicrons, VLDL IDL, HDL
E-4	35,000	Arg	Arg	Liver, peripheral tissues	Chylomicrons, VLDL IDL, HDL

Fig. 1.12 Apoprotein E's.

Fig. 1.13 Relative frequency of genotypes of apoprotein E's.

RELATIVE FREQUENCY OF GENOTYPES OF APOPROTEIN E'S

GENOTYPE	FREQUENCY (%)
E-3/E-3	60
E-3/E-4	22
E-3/E-2	12
E-4/E-4	3
E-4/E-2	2
E-2/E-2	1

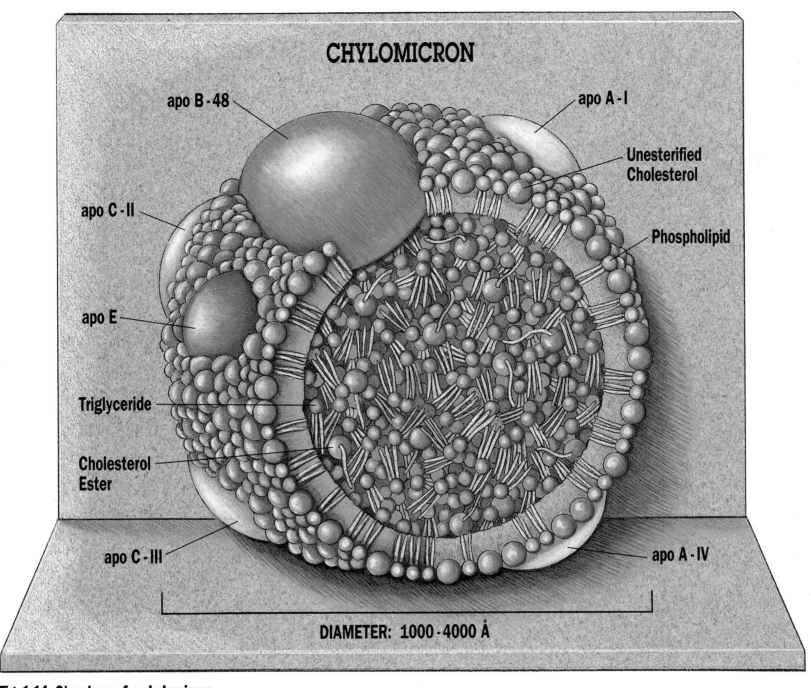

Fig. 1.14 Structure of a chylomicron.

apo C's are synthesized in the liver; in the circulation, they are carried on chylomicrons, VLDL, IDL, and HDL (Fig. 1.11). The three isoforms of apo E (E-2, E-3, E-4) each have a molecular weight of 35,000 daltons, and they differ only by the amino acids at positions 112 and 158 (Fig. 1.12). They are synthesized mainly in the liver, but small amounts can be made by other tissues. The apo E's are found in serum on chylomicrons, VLDL, IDL, and HDL. Every person inherits two isoforms of apo E — one from each parent. Consequently, six different genotypes are possible, and their relative frequencies in the general population are shown in Figure 1.13.

CHYLOMICRONS

The transport of cholesterol from the intestine to the liver occurs through lipoproteins called chylomicrons. These lipoproteins, which are synthesized in intestinal mucosal cells, are composed largely of triglycerides derived from dietary fat. Structurally, chylomicrons have a large nonpolar core consisting mostly of triglycerides and small amounts of cholesterol esters; its diameter ranges from 1000 to 4000 Å (Fig. 1.14). Several apoproteins are found in the surface covering. The major structural apoprotein of chylomicrons is apo B-48, which apparently is required for their synthesis. Apoproteins of the A series (A-I, A-II, and A-IV) also are secreted with chylomicrons. As chylomicrons enter the plasma, they

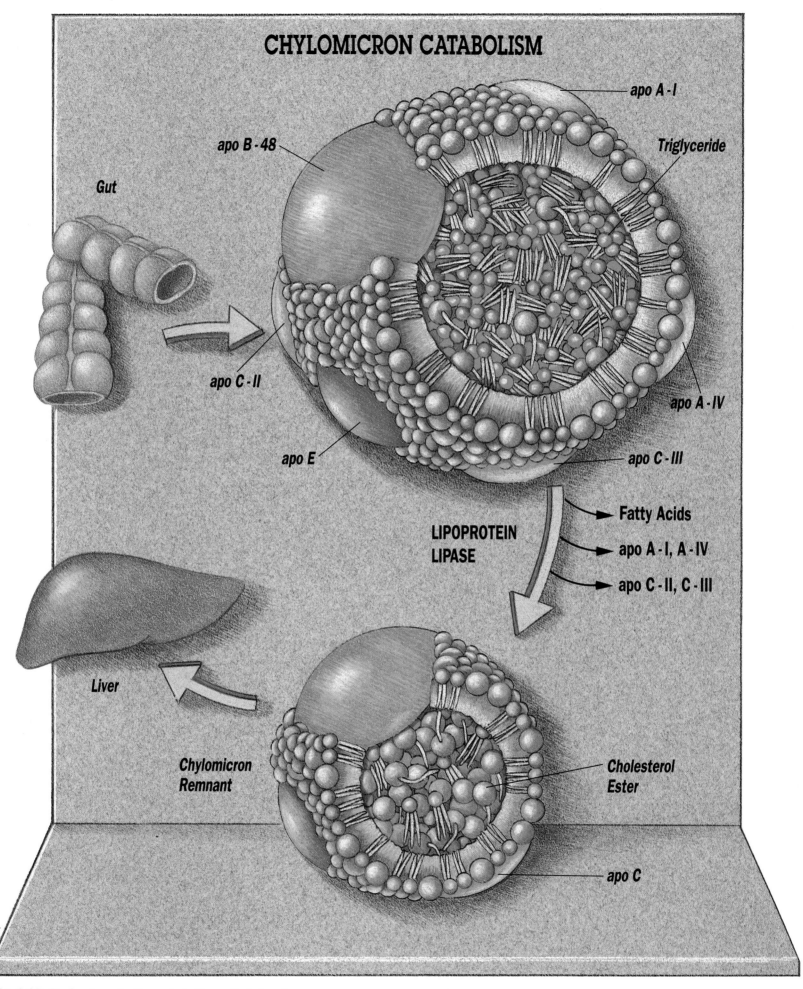

Fig. 1.15 Basic steps in the catabolism of chylomicrons.

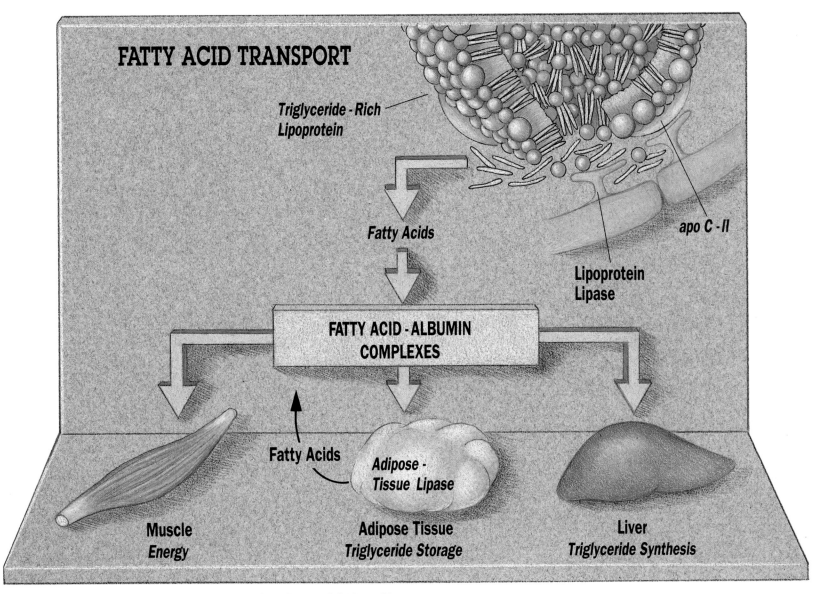

FATTY ACID TRANSPORT

Triglyceride - Rich Lipoprotein

apo C - II

Fatty Acids

Lipoprotein Lipase

FATTY ACID - ALBUMIN COMPLEXES

Fatty Acids

Adipose - Tissue Lipase

Muscle
Energy

Adipose Tissue
Triglyceride Storage

Liver
Triglyceride Synthesis

Fig. 1.16 Fatty - acid transport and the possible fates of fatty acids.

acquire apo E and the apo C's that are needed for their catabolism.

The basic steps in the catabolism of chylomicrons are presented in Figure 1.15. These lipoproteins are secreted first into the lymph and then enter the systemic circulation through the thoracic duct. As they pass into the peripheral circulation, they come into contact with the enzyme lipoprotein lipase, which is located on the surface of capillary endothelial cells. This enzyme hydrolyzes the triglycerides of chylomicrons, releasing free fatty acids into the circulation, along with apo A's and apo C's. After most of the triglycerides have been hydrolyzed, a residual lipoprotein — called a *chylomicron remnant* —returns

to the circulation. Containing mainly cholesterol esters in its core, this remnant lipoprotein is removed rapidly by the liver. Thus, during catabolism of chylomicrons, the fatty acids of dietary triglycerides are released into the peripheral circulation. This is in contrast to dietary cholesterol, which terminates in the liver as cholesterol esters with chylomicron remnants.

FATTY-ACID TRANSPORT

When triglyceride-rich lipoproteins, such as chylomicrons, interact with lipoprotein lipase, fatty acids are released from triglycerides (Fig. 1.16). Lipoprotein lipase is activated by apo C-II. The fatty

acids released during lipolysis immediately bind to circulating albumin and thereby are held in solution. The fatty acids can have three fates:

1. They can be taken up by muscle (and other tissues) and can be utilized for energy.
2. They can be taken up by adipose tissue where they are resynthesized into triglycerides for storage. When needed for fuel, these triglycerides undergo lipolysis by adipose-tissue lipase, and fatty acids again are released into the circulation.
3. They can be taken up by the liver where they serve as a source of fuel or can be resynthesized into triglycerides,

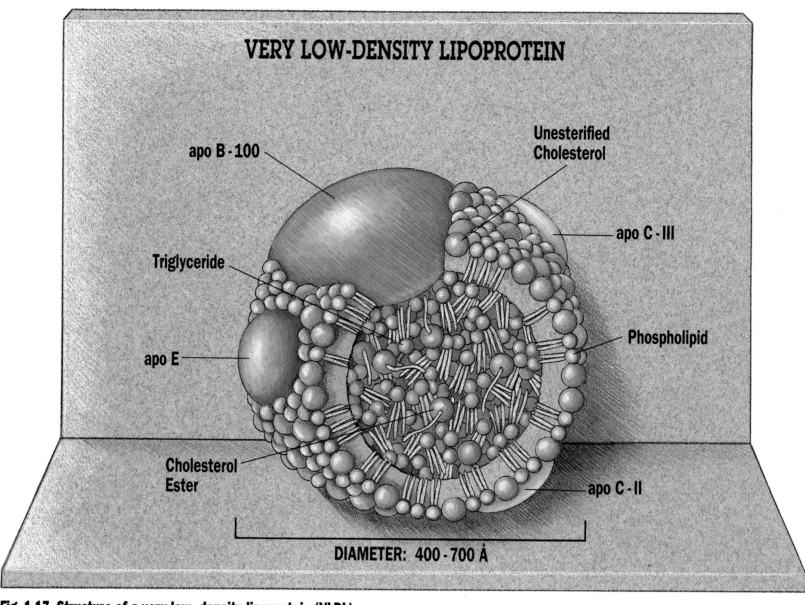

VERY LOW-DENSITY LIPOPROTEIN

apo B-100

Unesterified Cholesterol

Triglyceride

apo C-III

apo E

Phospholipid

Cholesterol Ester

apo C-II

DIAMETER: 400-700 Å

Fig. 1.17 Structure of a very low-density lipoprotein (VLDL).

which are used in the formation of hepatic triglyceride-rich lipoproteins.

VERY LOW-DENSITY LIPOPROTEINS

The major lipoprotein synthesized by the liver is the very low-density lipoprotein (VLDL). This triglyceride-rich lipoprotein is smaller than the chylomicron, its diameter ranging from 400 to 700 Å (Fig. 1.17). Its major structural apoprotein is apo B-100, but it also contains apo E and the apo C's (C-I, C-II, C-III). The major lipid component of the nonpolar core of VLDL is triglyceride, but cholesterol ester also is present. Besides the apoproteins, the surface coat contains unesterified cholesterol and phospholipids.

The basic steps in the synthesis of VLDL in the liver are presented in Fig-

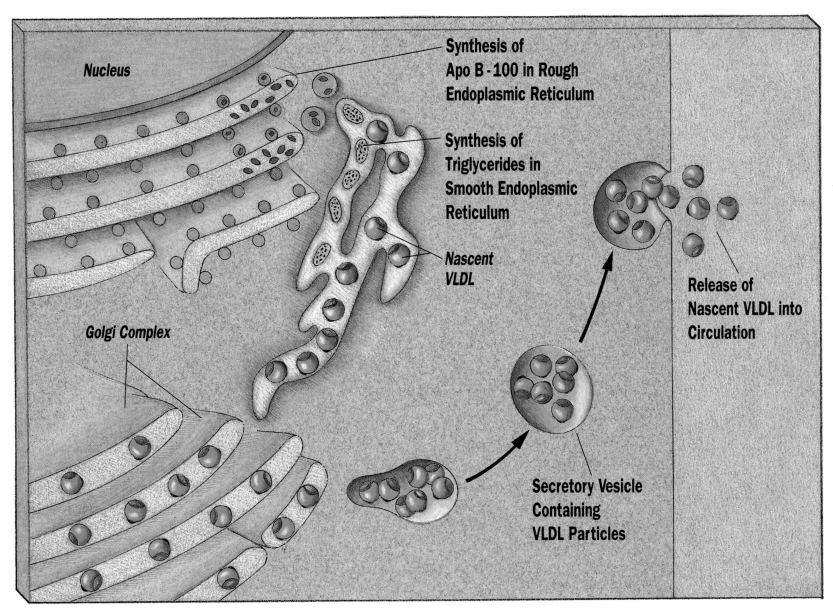

Fig. 1.18 Basic steps in the synthesis of VLDL.

ure 1.18. Apo B-100 is synthesized in ribosomes of the rough endoplasmic reticulum (RER). The triglyceride component of the lipoproteins, along with small amounts of cholesterol ester, is synthesized by membrane-bound enzymes located in the smooth endoplasmic reticulum (SER). As apo B-100 (and possibly apo E) migrate toward the SER, they join with triglyceride and cholesterol esters at the junction of the RER and the SER, and nascent VLDL particles are formed. The lipoprotein particles pass through the SER to the Golgi apparatus where secretory vesicles that contain large numbers of VLDL particles bud off and migrate to the surface of the cell. These vesicles then fuse with the membrane of the cell's surface and release nascent VLDL particles into the circulation.

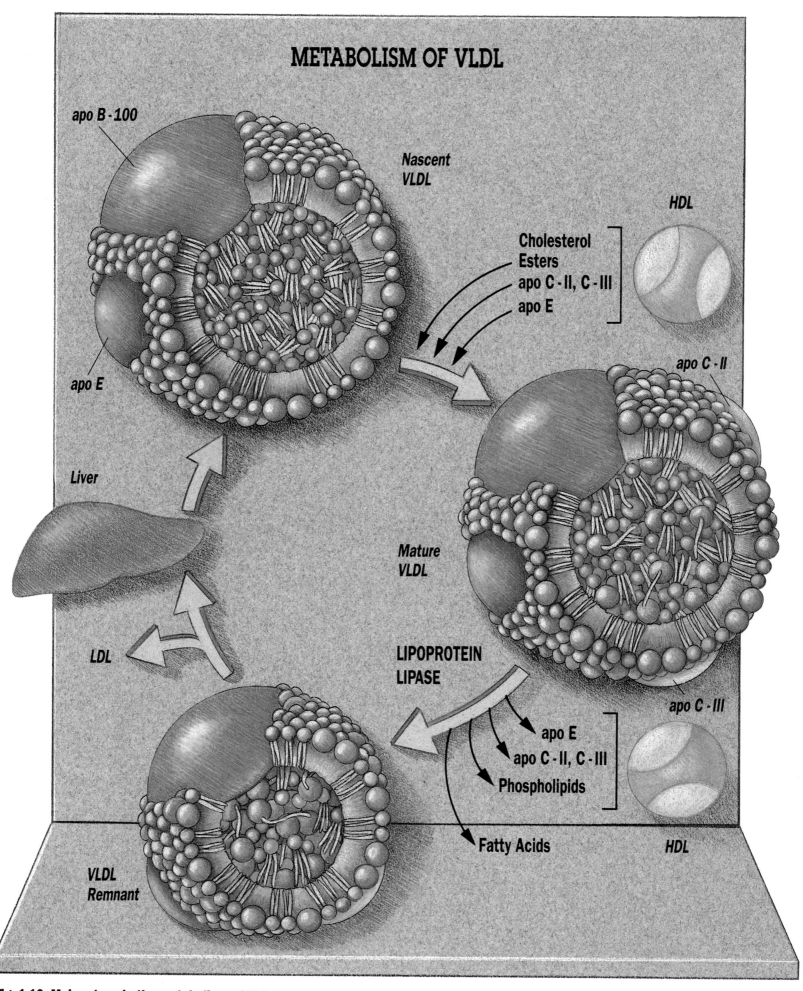

METABOLISM OF VLDL

apo B - 100

apo E

Nascent VLDL

HDL

Cholesterol Esters
apo C - II, C - III
apo E

apo C - II

Liver

Mature VLDL

LDL

LIPOPROTEIN LIPASE

apo C - III

apo E
apo C - II, C - III
Phospholipids

Fatty Acids

HDL

VLDL Remnant

Fig. 1.19 Major steps in the metabolism of VLDL.

The major steps in the metabolism of VLDL are outlined in Figure 1.19. As indicated above, the immediate lipoprotein secreted by the liver is nascent VLDL. The core of this particle consists almost exclusively of triglycerides; very little cholesterol ester is present. The surface coat of nascent VLDL contains apo B-100 and possibly apo E. As nascent VLDL circulate, they are transformed into mature VLDL. This transformation occurs by the acquisition of cholesterol esters and apoproteins C-II and C-III, and perhaps more apo E, all of which are transferred from high-density lipoproteins (HDL). Mature VLDL interact with lipoprotein lipase on the surface of capillary endothelial cells, and fatty acids are released into the circulation. Moreover, phospholipids, most apo C's, and some apo E's leave the surface coat of VLDL and are transferred to HDL. Remnant lipoproteins (VLDL remnants), produced from VLDL by lipoprotein lipase, are returned to the circulation. The core of VLDL remnants is enriched in cholesterol esters, both relatively and absolutely, because of hydrolysis of triglycerides and acquisition of cholesterol esters from HDL.

VLDL remnants can have two fates: they can be taken up by the liver or transformed into low-density lipoproteins (LDL) (Fig. 1.20). Normally, 60% to 70% of VLDL remnants are removed directly from the circulation by liver cells, apparently through the mediation of specific receptors located on the surface of these cells. One type of hepatic receptor is the LDL receptor (so named because it was first shown to clear LDL from the circulation); these receptors are concentrated in specific regions of the cell surface called coated pits. LDL receptors recognize both apo B-100 and apo E, and hence some investigators have called them B/E receptors. VLDL remnants also might be cleared by other receptors that recognize chylomicron remnants; the nature of these alternate receptors, however, has not been determined. VLDL remnants that are not removed by the liver seemingly can interact with hepatic triglyceride lipase, an enzyme located on the surface of liver cells. This enzyme can hydrolyze the remaining triglycerides of VLDL remnants, producing cholesterol-rich LDL. During the hydrolysis of triglycerides of VLDL remnants, fatty acids are released along with the remaining soluble apoproteins—apo E and small amounts of apo C's. Normally, 30% to 40% of all VLDL remnants are converted to LDL.

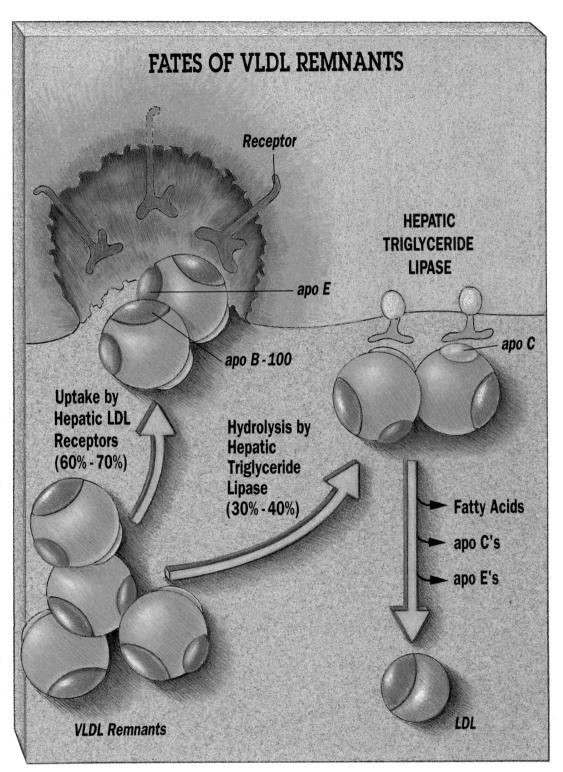

Fig. 1.20 Possible fates of VLDL remnants: uptake by the liver or transformation into low-density lipoproteins.

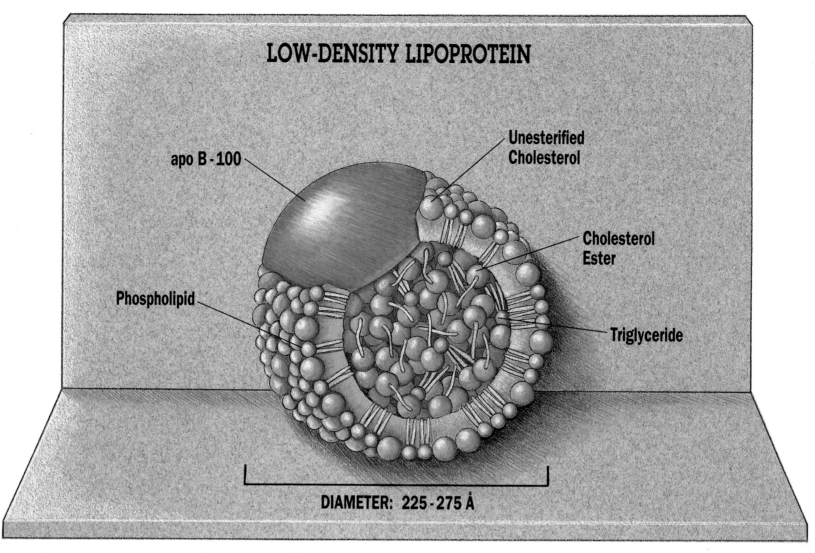

LOW-DENSITY LIPOPROTEIN

apo B - 100

Unesterified Cholesterol

Phospholipid

Cholesterol Ester

Triglyceride

DIAMETER: 225 - 275 Å

Fig. 1.21 Structure of a low-density lipoprotein (LDL).

LOW - DENSITY LIPOPROTEINS

The major cholesterol-carrying lipoprotein of plasma is the low-density lipoprotein (LDL). LDL consists of a lipid core composed almost entirely of cholesterol esters (approximately 1500 molecules in each LDL particle) (Fig. 1.21). The surface coat of LDL contains unesterified cholesterol and phospholipids, together with a single apoprotein, apo B-100. The diameter of the LDL particle ranges from 225 to 275 Å.

Fates of LDL. Circulating LDL can be removed from the bloodstream via either the liver or extrahepatic tissues (Fig. 1.22). Current estimates indicate that approximately 75% of serum LDL is cleared by the liver, with the remaining 25% by extrahepatic tissues. Uptake of LDL by either the liver or extrahepatic tissues can occur by both receptor and nonreceptor pathways. The latter are poorly defined, nonspecific pathways that clear plasma proteins in general. Apparently, two-thirds to three-fourths of the circulating pool of LDL is cleared by receptor pathways, whereas one-fourth to one-third is removed via nonreceptor pathways. On average, 30% to 40% of the total plasma pool of LDL is removed each day.

Receptor-Mediated Clearance of LDL. Pathways for uptake and degradation of LDL at the cellular level are shown in Figure 1.23. LDL receptors are transport-ed to the surface of cells, and from there they migrate to special regions on the cell surface called coated pits, where they aggregate and wait for LDL particles to arrive. When the LDL receptors bind to circulating LDL (or VLDL remnants), the receptor-ligand complexes are internalized into lysosomes. Following internalization, receptors disassociate from LDL and the former are recycled to the surface of the cell to be used again. The cholesterol esters of LDL are hydrolyzed to unesterified cholesterol, and apo B-100 is degraded to amino acids. The unesterified cholesterol derived from cholesterol esters can have several fates: It can serve as a constituent for cell membranes, it can

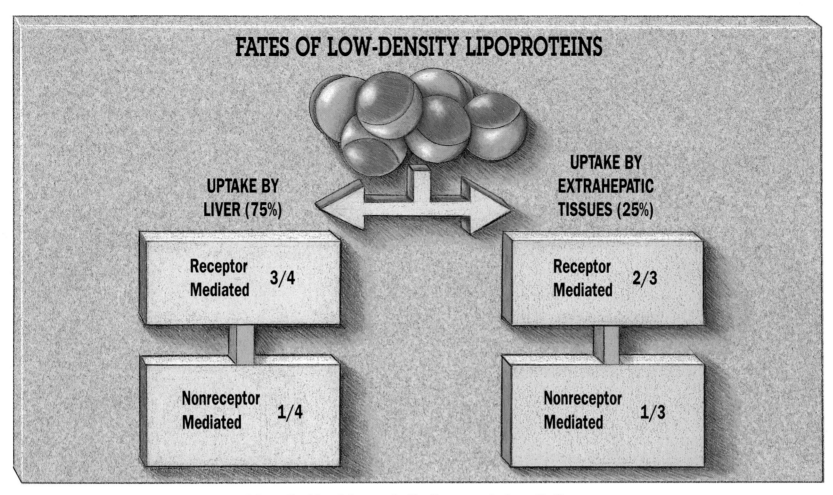

Fig. 1.22 Possible fates of LDL: removal from the bloodstream via the liver or extrahepatic tissues.

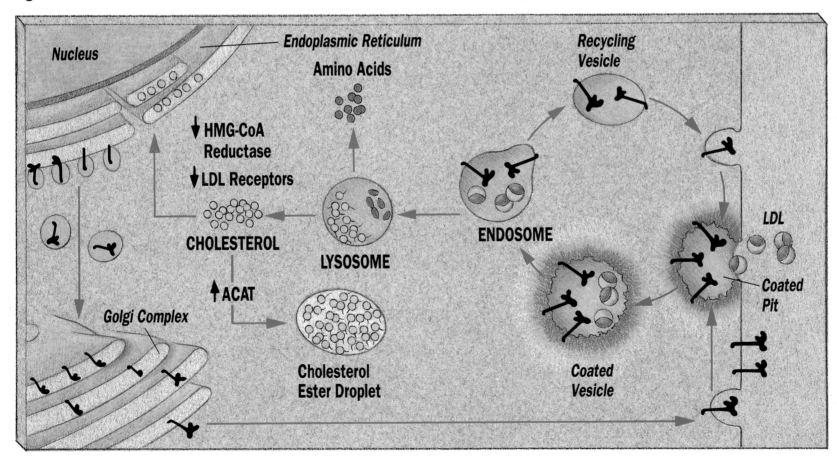

Fig. 1.23 Receptor-mediated clearance of LDL: pathways for uptake and degradation of LDL at the cellular level.

LDL RECEPTOR

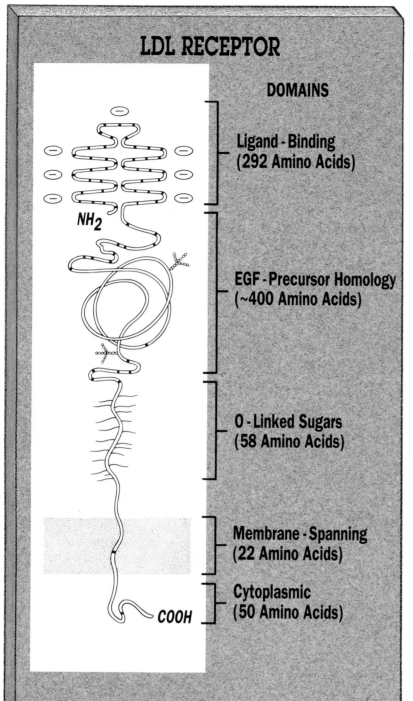

DOMAINS

Ligand - Binding
(292 Amino Acids)

EGF - Precursor Homology
(~400 Amino Acids)

O - Linked Sugars
(58 Amino Acids)

Membrane - Spanning
(22 Amino Acids)

Cytoplasmic
(50 Amino Acids)

REGULATION OF LDL-RECEPTOR SYNTHESIS

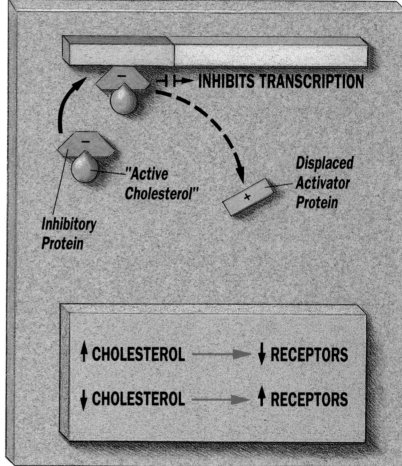

Fig. 1.24 Structure of the LDL receptor showing its functional domains. (Adapted from Brown and Goldstein, 1986)

Fig. 1.25 Postulated mechanism for regulation of LDL - receptor synthesis.

be reesterified into cholesterol ester for storage, or it can leave the cell. In the case of liver cells, cholesterol can exit into bile on the way to final excretion in stools. The amount of cholesterol entering the cell also regulates the activity of HMG-CoA reductase and the rate of synthesis of LDL receptors (see below).

Structure of the LDL Receptor. The LDL receptor is a molecule of molecular weight 120,000 containing approximately 820 amino acids. In addition, it contains a series of carbohydrate moieties that increase its molecular weight. The receptor has been shown to have several domains, each having unique functions (Fig. 1.24). The first domain, which has 292 amino acids, apparently is the portion required for binding LDL; it is located externally to the cell's plasma membrane. This domain has seven 40-amino-acid repeats, which may allow it to bind to more than one apoprotein at a time and to both apo B and apo E.

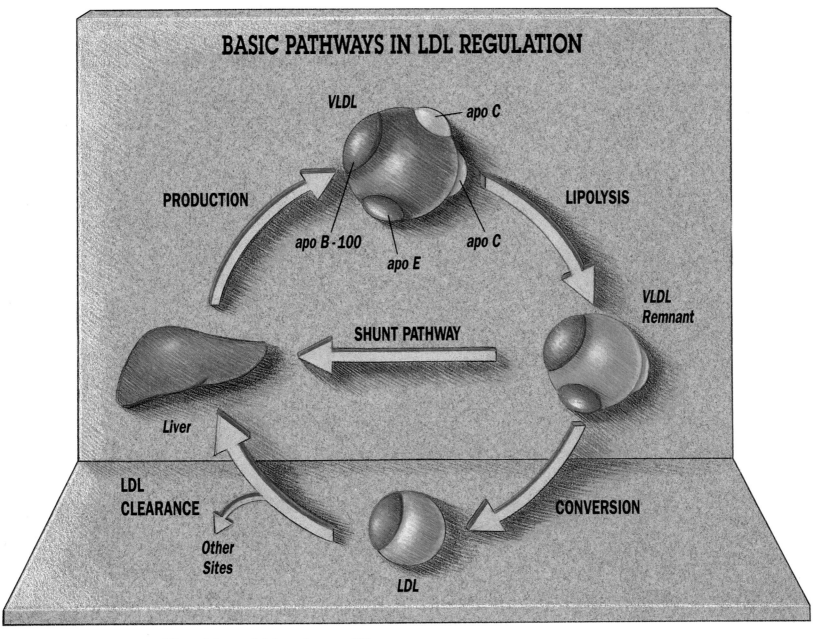

BASIC PATHWAYS IN LDL REGULATION

Fig. 1.26 Basic pathways of the origins and fates of serum LDL.

The second domain, which has approximately 400 amino acids, has homology to epidermal growth factor; the function of this long segment is unknown. The third domain, consisting of 58 amino acids, is the segment where the carbohydrate residues are linked. The next segment, having 22 amino acids, spans the cell's plasma membrane; it has a hydrophobic character. The fifth domain, which has 50 amino acids, projecting into the cytoplasm, may play an important role in causing the receptors to be clustered in coated pits.

Regulation of LDL-Receptor Synthesis. The number of LDL receptors synthesized by a cell is regulated by the amount of cholesterol in the cell. According to the postulated mechanism of receptor-synthesis regulation (Fig. 1.25), a small portion of cellular cholesterol appears to be converted into an "active" form, most likely an "oxy"-sterol, that more readily enters the cell's nucleus. This "active cholesterol" interacts with a regulatory protein or proteins, which in turn suppress the activity of the gene encoding for the LDL receptor by affecting the promoter region of the gene. When the cellular content of cholesterol increases, the number of receptors produced by the cell decreases; conversely, when the

cholesterol content declines, receptor number increases. This tightly controlled regulatory system functions to maintain the cellular content of cholesterol in a narrow optimal range.

General Regulation of Serum-LDL Levels. The basic pathways of the origins and fates of serum LDL are shown in Figure 1.26. The immediate precursor of LDL is the VLDL remnant, which in turn is derived from VLDL. The amount of LDL produced depends on two factors: (1) the quantity of VLDL produced by the liver and (2) the fraction of VLDL remnants removed directly by the liver. The latter is determined in part by the

HIGH-DENSITY LIPOPROTEIN

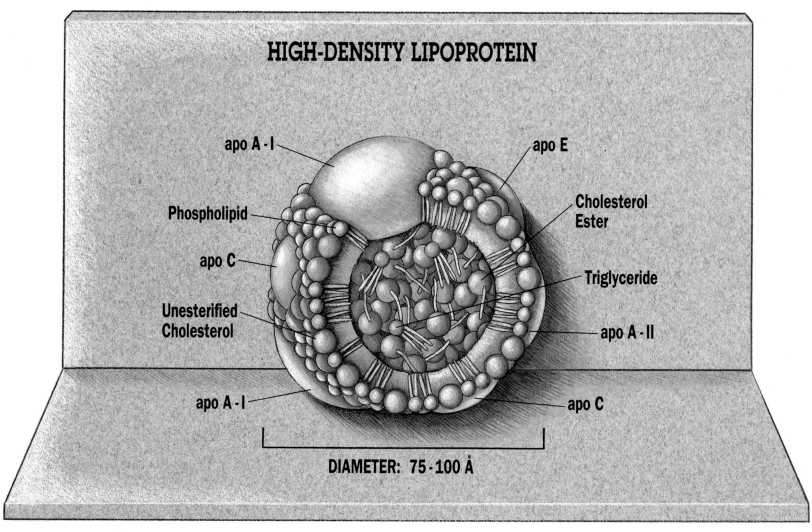

apo A - I

apo E

Phospholipid

Cholesterol Ester

apo C

Triglyceride

Unesterified Cholesterol

apo A - II

apo A - I

apo C

DIAMETER: 75 - 100 Å

Fig. 1.27 Structure of a high-density lipoprotein (HDL).

number of LDL receptors, since VLDL remnants can be removed by LDL receptors. The concentration of LDL also is determined by the rate of its removal from the circulation, either by the liver or by extrahepatic tissues. Again, LDL receptors are largely responsible for clearance of serum LDL. Thus, the number of LDL receptors is a key regulator of serum-LDL concentrations by affecting *both* the rate of formation and the rate of clearance of LDL.

HIGH - DENSITY LIPOPROTEINS

The final class of lipoproteins in the serum are the high-density lipoproteins (HDL). They are the smallest of the lipoproteins, having diameters in the range of 75 to 100 Å; and their lipid core is composed mainly of cholesterol esters (Fig. 1.27). The major apoproteins of HDL are apo A-I and A-II. Apo A-I is a monomer of molecular weight 28,000, whereas apo A-II is a dimer composed of two monomers linked by disulfide bonds; apo A-II is less water-soluble than apo

A-I and remains more tightly bound to the HDL particle. The surface coat of HDL also contains apo C's and apo E's, which can readily be transferred to triglyceride-rich lipoproteins (VLDL and chylomicrons).

Maturation of HDL. HDL is formed in a series of steps (Fig. 1.28). The first step is the secretion into serum of a precursor to HDL called nascent HDL. Both liver and small intestine synthesize nascent HDL. These particles, which are disc-shaped, consist of a phospholipid bilayer, within which reside apo A-I, apo A-II, and possibly apo E. Nascent HDL are good acceptors of unesterified cholesterol, which can come from either cell membranes of various tissues or the surface coats of other lipoproteins. When unesterified cholesterol reaches the surface of nascent HDL, it is transformed into cholesterol ester through the action of the enzyme lecithin–cholesterol acyltransferase (LCAT). This enzyme transfers a fatty acid from a lecithin molecule to cholesterol. As cholesterol esters begin to accumulate in HDL particles, they form a lipid core, transforming the disc-shaped particles into spheres. The smallest spherical form of HDL is named HDL_3. However, HDL_3 continues to acquire more unesterified cholesterol, which in turn is esterified through the action of LCAT, further enlarging the lipoprotein and thereby producing HDL_2. In normal serum, there are two or three HDL_3 particles for every one HDL_2 particle.

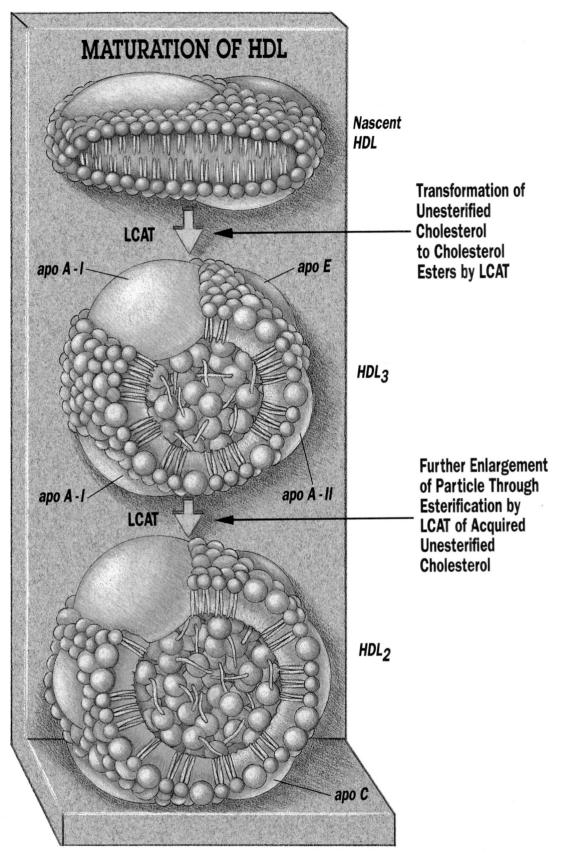

MATURATION OF HDL

Nascent HDL

LCAT

apo A-I

apo E

Transformation of Unesterified Cholesterol to Cholesterol Esters by LCAT

HDL_3

apo A-I

apo A-II

LCAT

Further Enlargement of Particle Through Esterification by LCAT of Acquired Unesterified Cholesterol

HDL_2

apo C

Fig. 1.28 Basic steps in the maturation of HDL.

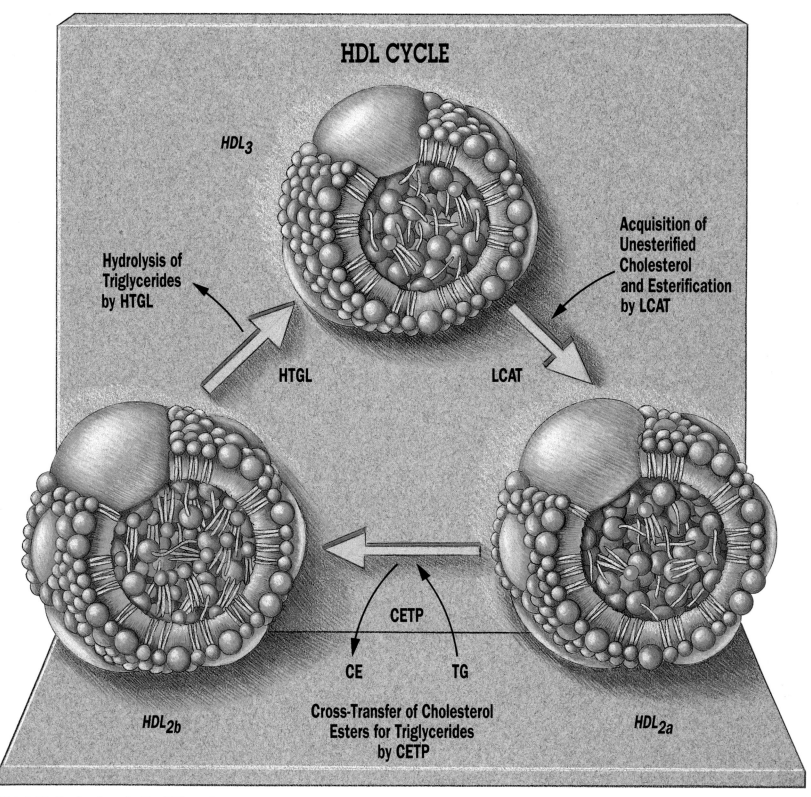

Fig. 1.29 Basic steps in the HDL cycle.

HDL Cycle. There appears to be an interconversion among the different forms of HDL (Fig. 1.29). First, HDL$_3$ is transformed into HDL$_{2a}$ by the acquisition of cholesterol esters. HDL$_{2a}$, in turn, is converted into HDL$_{2b}$ through the exchange of cholesterol esters for triglycerides. Triglycerides are derived from triglyceride-rich lipoproteins, which in exchange receive cholesterol esters from HDL. This cross-transfer reaction is mediated by a protein known as cholesterol-ester transfer protein (CETP). Finally, HDL$_{2b}$, which is enriched in triglycerides, is transformed back into HDL$_3$ by hydrolysis of its triglycerides, apparently through the action of hepatic triglyceride lipase (HTGL). This cycle may be important in the transfer of cholesterol from peripheral tissues to the liver, a process known as reverse cholesterol transport.

Reverse Cholesterol Transport. Cholesterol can only be degraded and excreted by the liver. Therefore, to remove excess cholesterol from peripheral tissues, cholesterol must be transported back to the liver. Figure 1.30 shows two mechanisms, and perhaps the major mechanisms, for reverse choles-

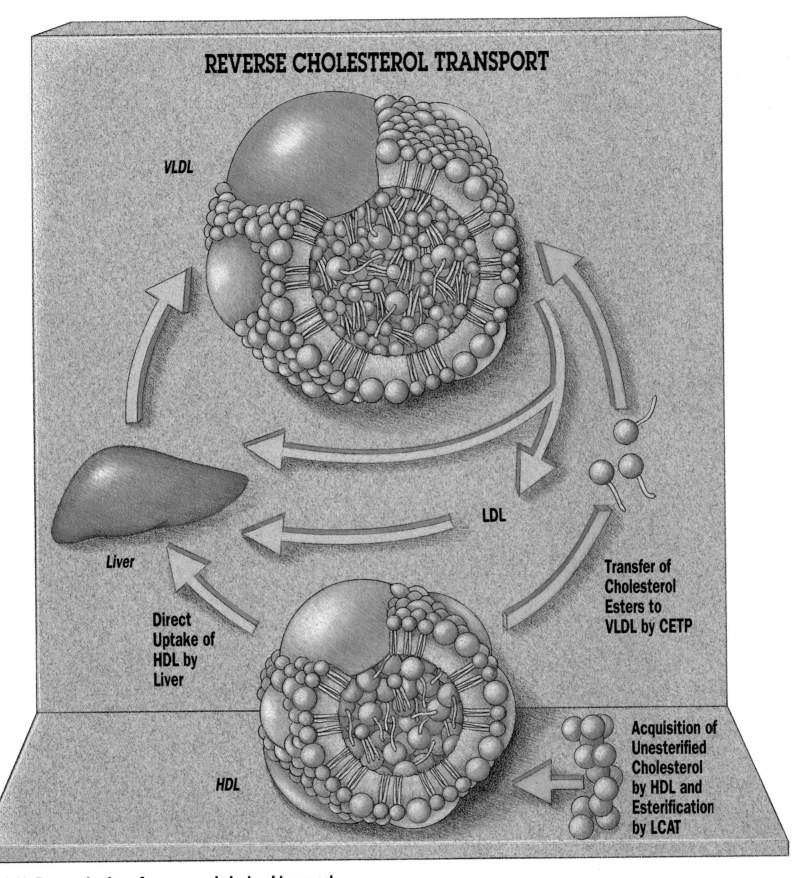

REVERSE CHOLESTEROL TRANSPORT

VLDL

Liver

LDL

Direct Uptake of HDL by Liver

Transfer of Cholesterol Esters to VLDL by CETP

HDL

Acquisition of Unesterified Cholesterol by HDL and Esterification by LCAT

Fig. 1.30 Two mechanisms for reverse cholesterol transport.

terol transport. In the first, unesterified cholesterol in the surface membranes of cells is transferred to HDL, and through the action of LCAT the cholesterol is esterified. A portion of HDL cholesterol ester is shuttled to VLDL by CETP. The cholesterol ester in VLDL can then be returned to the liver by direct uptake of VLDL remnants or after conversion of VLDL to LDL. By the second mechanism, whole HDL particles possibly can be removed intact by the liver. Although this second pathway remains somewhat conjectural, the first is well documented.

Fig. 1.31 Steps in atherogenesis.

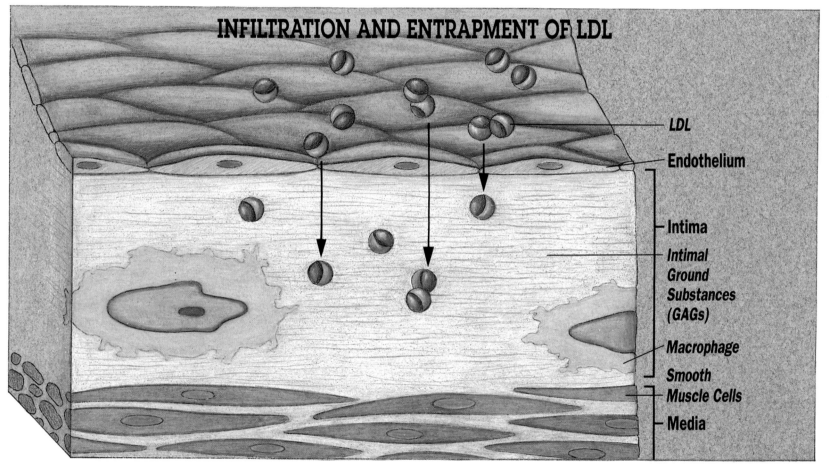

STEPS IN ATHEROGENESIS

INFILTRATION OF LDL INTO ARTERIAL WALL

ENTRAPMENT OF LDL IN ARTERIAL WALL

MODIFICATION OF LDL

UPTAKE OF MODIFIED LDL BY MACROPHAGES
Formation of foam cells
Formation of fatty streaks

CONVERSION OF FATTY STREAKS TO FIBROUS PLAQUES

INFILTRATION AND ENTRAPMENT OF LDL

- LDL
- Endothelium
- Intima
- Intimal Ground Substances (GAGs)
- Macrophage
- Smooth Muscle Cells
- Media

Fig. 1.32 Steps in atherogenesis: infiltration of LDL particles through endothelium of arterial wall into intimal layer where some are entrapped.

CHOLESTEROL AND ATHEROSCLEROSIS
STEPS IN ATHEROGENESIS

Serum cholesterol plays a key role in the development of atherosclerosis. Most investigators believe that the cholesterol carried in LDL is quantitatively the most atherogenic form of serum cholesterol. However, many workers believe that VLDL remnants also are atherogenic, and the basic mechanisms whereby VLDL remnants contribute to atherosclerosis probably are similar to those for LDL. The essential steps in atherogenesis are outlined in Figure 1.31. First, LDL (and/or VLDL remnants) filter into the arterial wall and become entrapped in the intima where they undergo chemical modification. This leads to the uptake of modified LDL by macrophages to produce foam cells. The accumulation of foam cells in the intima results in the formation of fatty streaks. The latter are gradually converted into fibrous plaques by a mechanism similar to scar formation. Finally, fibrous plaques can be transformed into complicated atherosclerotic lesions, which underly most clinical events. All of these steps are described in greater detail in the following sections.

Infiltration and Entrapment of LDL. Circulating LDL particles filter through the endothelium of the arterial wall and penetrate into the intimal layer (Fig. 1.32). This process may be accelerated by endothelial injury, which removes a natural barrier to the entrance of lipoproteins into the wall of the artery. A portion of LDL particles passes completely through the intimal layer and reenters the circulation through the vasa vasorum. However, a portion of LDL becomes entrapped in the intima.

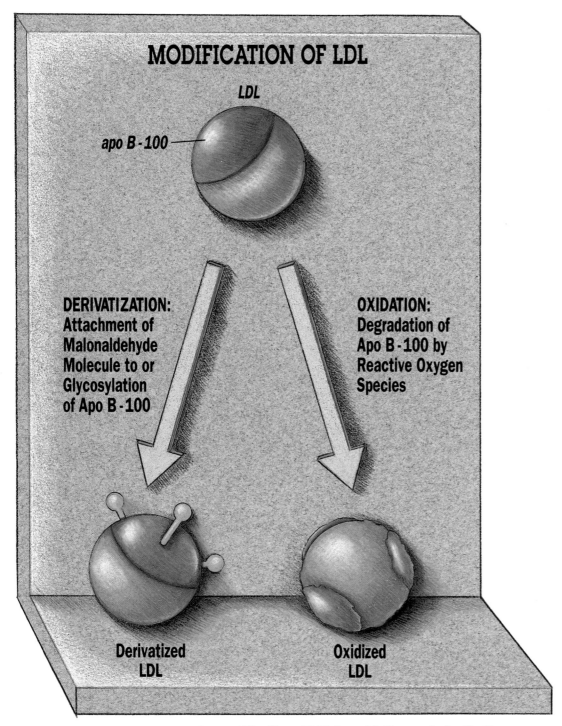

MODIFICATION OF LDL

LDL

apo B - 100

DERIVATIZATION:
Attachment of
Malonaldehyde
Molecule to or
Glycosylation
of Apo B - 100

OXIDATION:
Degradation of
Apo B - 100 by
Reactive Oxygen
Species

Derivatized
LDL

Oxidized
LDL

Fig. 1.33 Steps in atherogenesis: modification of LDL by oxidation or derivatization.

Entrapment is thought to occur through the interaction of LDL with components of the intimal ground substances, most likely glycoaminoglycans (GAGs), which appear to have a high affinity for the apo B-100 of LDL. The interaction of apo B-100 with GAGs, resulting in the trapping of LDL in the intima, represents a key first step in atherogenesis. It would appear that only lipoproteins containing apo B-100 (i.e., LDL, IDL, VLDL) have the potential to produce atherosclerosis. An exception may be cholesterol-rich chylomicron remnants that contain apo B-48. In contrast, HDL, which do not contain any form of apo B, are not atherogenic.

Modification of LDL. Once entrapped in the arterial intima, LDL begin to undergo modification (Fig. 1.33). Two types of modification have been identified; one of these is *oxidation.* Macrophages in the arterial wall are known to secrete superoxide, presumably as part of their phagocytic function. This superoxide can attack apo B-100 and oxidatively degrade it. As the apo B-100 is degraded, the LDL particle begins to lose its integrity, making it ripe for engulfment by macrophages. Alternatively, the apo B-100 of LDL can undergo *derivatization.* Several derivatives have been postulated. One of the more likely is the attachment of a mal-

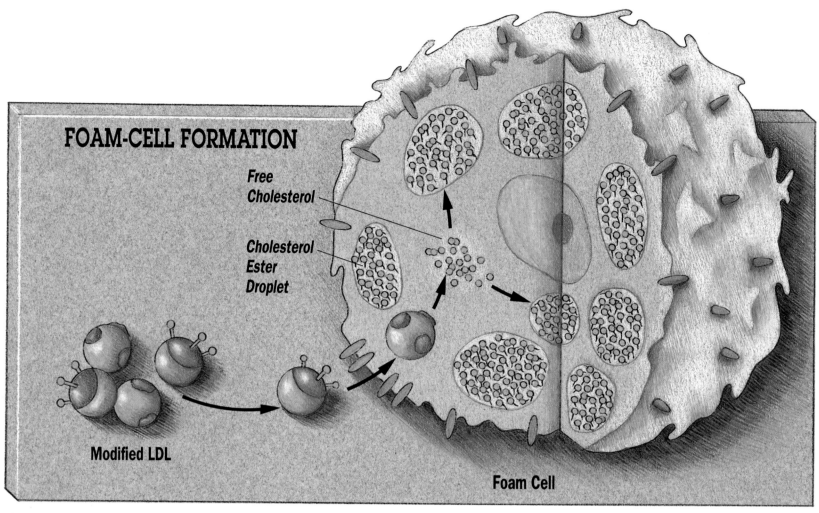

FOAM-CELL FORMATION

Free
Cholesterol

Cholesterol
Ester
Droplet

Modified LDL

Foam Cell

Fig. 1.34 Steps in atherogenesis: ingestion of modified LDL by macrophages initiating the formation of foam cells.

onaldehyde molecule to apo B, while another possibility is glycosylation of apo B. Like "oxidized" LDL, the "derivatized" LDL particles are subject to engulfment by macrophages.

Foam-Cell Formation. The foam cell is the hallmark of the atherosclerotic lesion. Most foam cells are currently thought to be derived from macrophages, although some may come from smooth muscle cells. The key step in the development of foam cells is the ingestion of modified LDL (Fig. 1.34). When normal LDL are taken up by the LDL-receptor pathway, the cholesterol released from LDL acts to inhibit the synthesis of new LDL receptors; therefore, excess cholesterol cannot accumulate in the cell. In other words, foam-cell formation seemingly does not occur through the LDL-receptor pathway. However, macrophages also possess receptors for modified LDL. When LDL enter the cell through this mechanism, there is no feedback control on the for-

mation of new receptors; thus, modified-LDL receptors continue to take up modified-LDL particles regardless of how much cholesterol accumulates in cells. This leads to the formation of many large droplets of cholesterol ester that give the cell a foamy appearance, hence the name *foam* cell.

STAGES OF ATHEROSCLEROSIS

Three stages of the atherosclerotic plaque are recognized: (1) the fatty streak, (2) the fibrous plaque, and (3) the complicated lesion (Fig. 1.35). The *fatty streak* is characterized by the accumulation of foam cells and intercellular lipid in the intima of an artery. Fatty streaks do not produce significant obstruction of the arterial lumen. Many workers believe that fatty streaks are transformed into the next stage of the atherosclerotic lesion, the *fibrous plaque*. A direct link between the fatty

streak and the fibrous plaque almost certainly exists within the coronary arteries, whereas evidence for a linkage is less strong for other arteries, such as the aorta. In the latter, fatty streaks and fibrous plaques do not necessarily occur in the same areas. The fibrous plaque is a proliferative lesion in which a fibrous cap covers a lipid core Smooth muscle cells are present that produce fibrous connective tissue containing ground substance, collagen fibers, and reticulum fibrils. Sometimes small mural thrombi may be found on the surface of fibrous plaques. The lipid core is lined by foam cells that surround an amorphous extracellular accumulation of cholesterol esters. The third stage of plaque development is a *complicated lesion*. This lesion can manifest calcification, hemorrhage, ulceration (rupture), and thrombosis. The complicated lesion frequently underlies the acute clinical event of arterial occlusion.

STAGES OF ATHEROSCLEROSIS

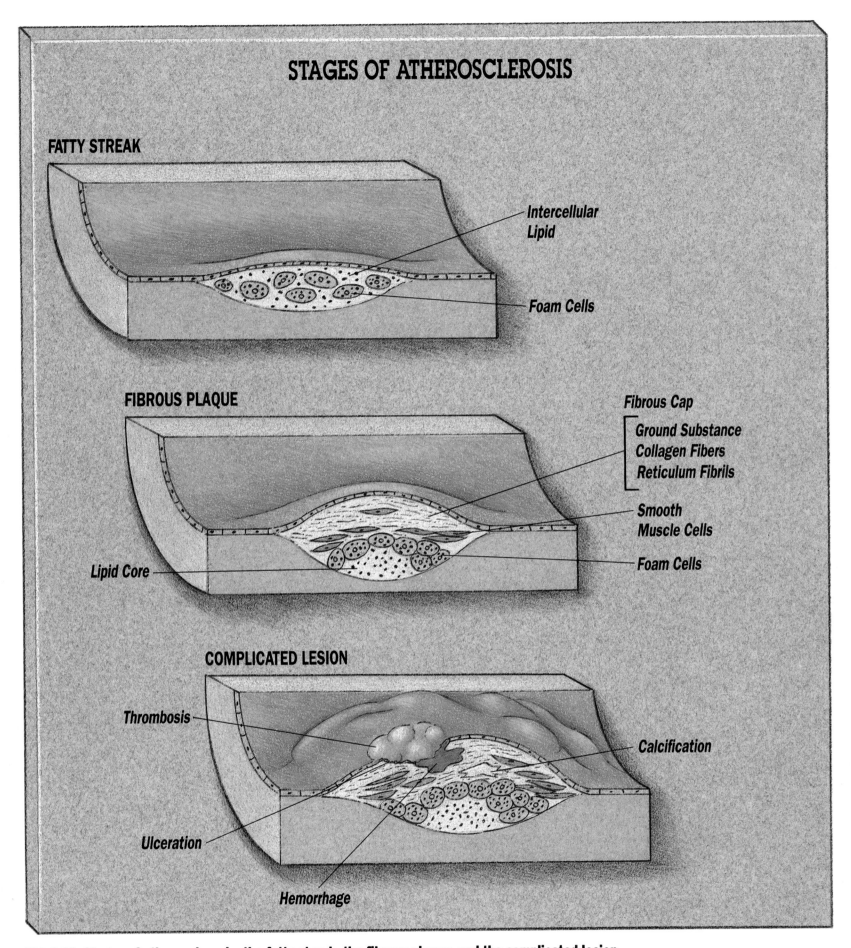

FATTY STREAK

Intercellular Lipid

Foam Cells

FIBROUS PLAQUE

Fibrous Cap
Ground Substance
Collagen Fibers
Reticulum Fibrils

Smooth Muscle Cells

Foam Cells

Lipid Core

COMPLICATED LESION

Thrombosis

Calcification

Ulceration

Hemorrhage

Fig. 1.35 Stages of atherosclerosis: the fatty streak, the fibrous plaque, and the complicated lesion.

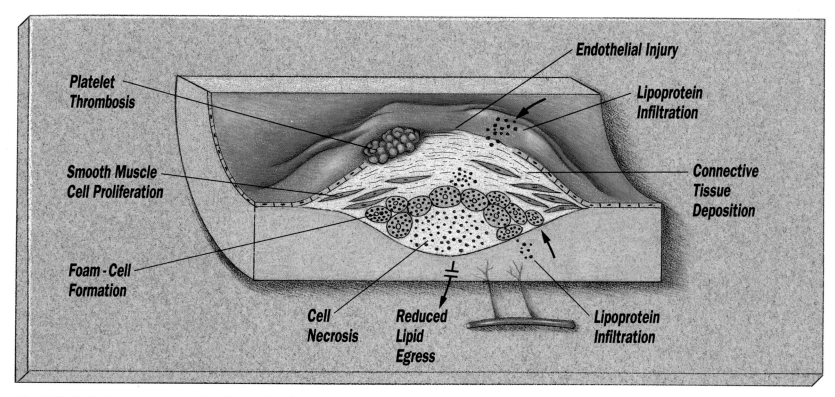

Fig. 1.36 Pathologic processes leading to the development of an atherosclerotic plaque.

Fig. 1.37 Effects of risk factors on atherogenesis.

EFFECTS OF RISK FACTORS ON ATHEROGENESIS

RISK FACTOR	EFFECTS
Increased LDL, IDL, VLDL	Increased lipoprotein infiltration into arterial wall
Decreased HDL	Decreased cholesterol egress from arterial wall
Hypertension	Enhanced lipoprotein infiltration into arterial wall Arterial endothelial injury
Cigarette smoking	Arterial endothelial injury Arterial-wall hypoxia Thrombosis
Diabetes mellitus	Multiple effects (e.g., hyperlipidemia, reduced HDL, endothelial injury)

PATHOGENESIS OF ATHEROSCLEROTIC PLAQUE

The various pathologic processes leading to the formation of an atherosclerotic plaque are summarized in Figure 1.36. Lipoprotein infiltration through either the luminal endothelium or the vasa vasorum into the arterial wall appears to be the first step. Some lipoproteins are trapped in the intimal ground substance, modified, and ingested by macrophages to produce foam cells. The infiltration of lipoproteins may be accelerated by endothelial injury, which removes a natural barrier to the entrance of lipoproteins into the wall of an artery. Platelet thrombi may form on the exposed surface beneath the area of endothelial injury. Both foam cells and platelets release growth factors that cause proliferation of smooth muscle cells and deposition of connective tissue elements. Engorgement of foam cells with lipids (and perhaps local hypoxia) seemingly causes cellular necrosis and release of cholesterol esters from foam cells to produce the lipid core. Destruction of the vasa vasorum may interfere with egress of lipids from the plaque. All these changes set the stage for the final complications: hemorrhage into the plaque causing plaque rupture, thrombosis, and vascular occlusion.

EFFECTS OF RISK FACTORS ON ATHEROGENESIS

Several risk factors for CHD appear to promote the development of atherosclerosis: (1) increased cholesterol in LDL, IDL, and VLDL, (2) low levels of HDL-cholesterol, (3) hypertension, (4) cigarette smoking, and (5) diabetes mellitus (Fig. 1.37). The precise means

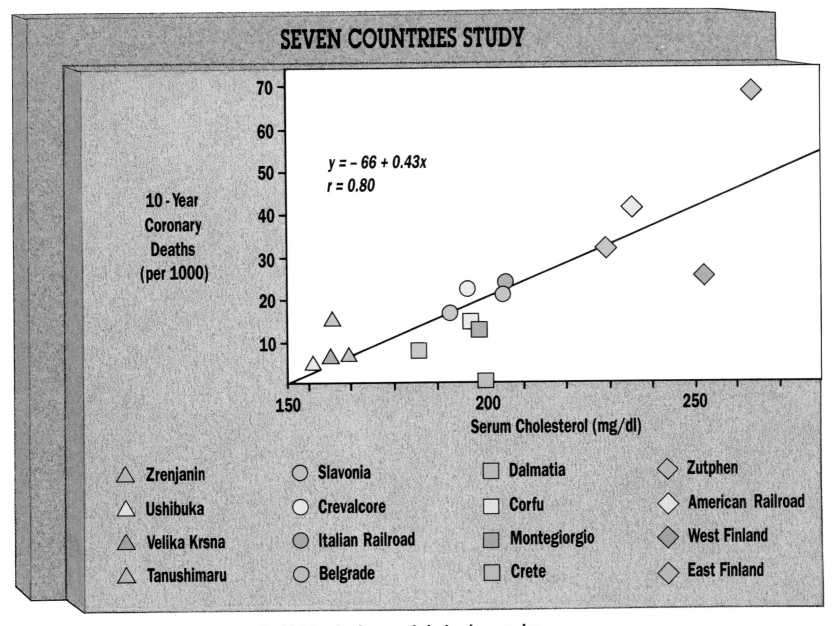

SEVEN COUNTRIES STUDY

$y = -66 + 0.43x$
$r = 0.80$

10-Year Coronary Deaths (per 1000)

Serum Cholesterol (mg/dl)

△ Zrenjanin   ○ Slavonia   □ Dalmatia   ◇ Zutphen

△ Ushibuka   ○ Crevalcore   □ Corfu   ◇ American Railroad

△ Velika Krsna   ○ Italian Railroad   □ Montegiorgio   ◇ West Finland

△ Tanushimaru   ○ Belgrade   □ Crete   ◇ East Finland

Fig. 1.38 Epidemiologic evidence supporting high levels of serum cholesterol as a major risk factor for CHD : the Seven Countries Study.

whereby each of these factors accelerates atherosclerosis are not fully understood, but several mechanisms have been postulated. Increased levels of LDL, IDL, and VLDL are associated with enhanced filtration of lipoproteins into the arterial wall, leading to intercellular accumulation of lipids and foam-cell formation. A low level of HDL-cholesterol may interfere with the normal egress of cholesterol from the arterial wall. Hypertension probably increases the rate of infiltration of lipoproteins into the arterial wall by enhanced lateral pressure, and increased sheer forces may cause endothelial injury. Injury to the endothelium also may result from the toxic products of cigarette smoke; these substances produce hypoxia in the arterial wall, which may cause cellular necrosis and initiate events leading to hemorrhage into plaques and arterial thrombosis. Finally, diabetes mellitus

may promote development of atherosclerosis by multiple mechanisms: hyperlipidemia, reduced HDL levels, modification of lipoproteins in the arterial wall, endothelial injury, stimulation of cellular proliferation, increased secretion of fibrous connective tissue, or acceleration of aging of arterial cells. The multiple effects of different risk factors set the stage for a synergistic interaction of risk factors that greatly accelerates the development of atherosclerosis.

CHOLESTEROL AND CORONARY HEART DISEASE

EVIDENCE SUPPORTING A RELATIONSHIP

Epidemiologic Evidence. Three types of epidemiologic evidence support the concept that high levels of serum cholesterol are a major risk factor for CHD. One type of evidence is derived from *between-*

countries studies. This is illustrated by the Seven Countries Studies carried out by Ancel Keys and associates in the 1960's. These workers compared levels of total cholesterol to rates of CHD in several different populations in seven countries (Fig. 1.38). In those countries having the highest cholesterol levels (e.g., Finland), rates of CHD likewise were highest; in contrast, countries having low levels of serum cholesterol (e.g., Japan and Crete) also had low CHD rates. Countries with intermediate cholesterol levels had intermediate rates of CHD. Although other factors undoubtedly influenced the development of CHD in these different populations, there was overall a high correlation between cholesterol levels and CHD rates, a correlation strongly implicating elevated serum cholesterol in the causation of CHD.

A second type of epidemiologic evidence comes from *migration studies.* The

Fig. 1.39 Epidemiologic evidence supporting the high cholesterol – CHD connection: comparison of cholesterol levels and CHD rates in Japanese living in Japan, Hawaii, and San Francisco.

COMPARISON OF CHOLESTEROL LEVELS AND CHD RATES IN JAPANESE LIVING IN JAPAN, HAWAII, AND SAN FRANCISCO

	JAPAN	HAWAII	SAN FRANCISCO
SERUM CHOLESTEROL (mg/dl)	181	218	228
CHD RATE (per 1000)	25.4	34.7	44.6

Fig. 1.40 Epidemiologic evidence supporting high total cholesterol as a powerful risk factor for CHD: follow-up survey of 360,000 men screened for MRFIT.

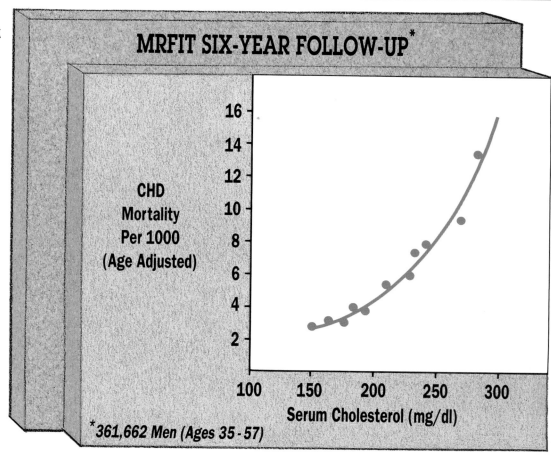

MRFIT SIX-YEAR FOLLOW-UP*

CHD Mortality Per 1000 (Age Adjusted)

Serum Cholesterol (mg/dl)

*361,662 Men (Ages 35 - 57)

most notable of these is a comparison of CHD rates in Japanese living in Japan, Honolulu, and San Francisco. The comparison showed that migration from Japan resulted in a progressive rise in cholesterol levels and a corresponding increase in CHD rates (Fig. 1.39). These data add further support to the cholesterol–CHD connection.

The third category of epidemiologic evidence is a series of *studies within a single country*. Many such studies have been carried out in several countries throughout the world. The best known investigation of this type in the United States is the Framingham Heart Study,

in which a large portion of the population of Framingham, Massachusetts, has been followed for many years. The results of this study have revealed a strong correlation between serum cholesterol levels and rates of CHD, particularly at higher levels of cholesterol. A few years ago the results from Framingham were combined with those of four other large surveys in the United States, and this "pooling" project again revealed a strong relationship between cholesterol levels and CHD rates. Finally, perhaps the best comparison is that of a follow-up survey of 361,662 men screened for the Multiple Risk Factor

Intervention Trial (MRFIT). This survey revealed a strong, positive curvilinear relationship between cholesterol levels at initial screening and subsequent CHD mortality (Fig. 1.40); these results leave little doubt that high total cholesterol is a powerful risk factor for CHD.

Experimental - Animal Evidence. The first evidence that serum cholesterol levels are linked to CHD was obtained in laboratory animals. Feeding of cholesterol to rabbits induces marked hypercholesterolemia and atherosclerosis. Subsequent studies have shown that many laboratory animals are susceptible to hypercholesterolemia-induced

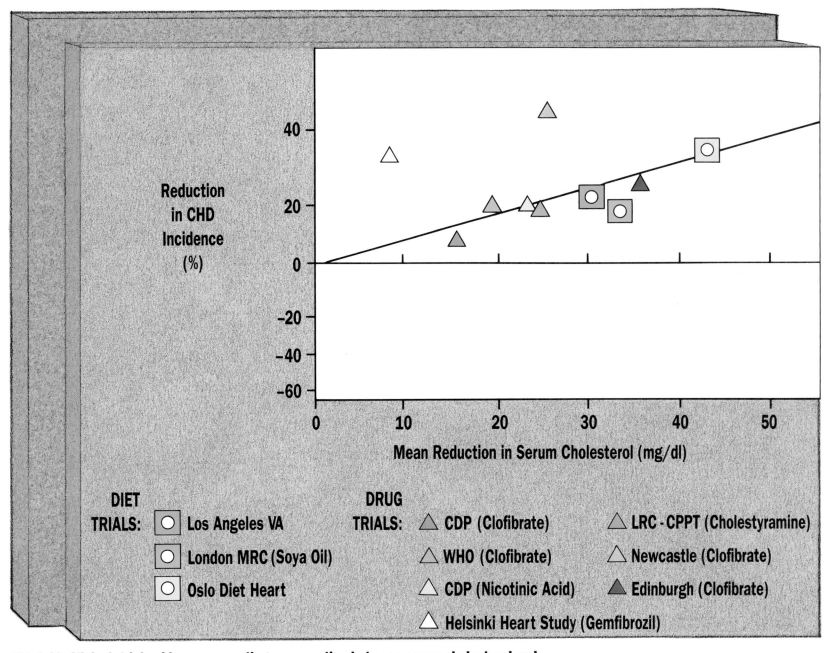

Fig. 1.41 Clinical - trial evidence supporting a connection between serum cholesterol and CHD: therapeutic lowering of cholesterol levels in hypercholesterolemic patients reduces risk for CHD.

atherosclerosis. In some instances (e.g., rabbits, chickens, and certain primates), hypercholesterolemia can be induced by feeding excess dietary cholesterol; in others (e.g., rats, dogs), dietary cholesterol alone will not cause marked hypercholesterolemia, but when elevated cholesterol levels are induced by other means, atherosclerosis will develop. Recently, genetic forms of hypercholesterolemia have been identified in different species, and these are uniformly accompanied by marked atherosclerosis. The many findings in laboratory animals provide a strong mechanistic connection between serum cholesterol and atherosclerosis.

Genetic Hyperlipidemias and Atherosclerosis in Humans. Several different genetic forms of hyperlipidemia have been identified in man, and many of these are accompanied by premature CHD. (These disorders are discussed in more detail in Unit 2.) The significance of these disorders is that they can produce premature CHD in the absence of other coronary risk factors. Thus, they provide strong evidence that hyperlipidemia, particularly elevated serum total cholesterol, is a powerful independent risk factor for CHD.

Clinical-Trial Evidence. Still another type of evidence linking serum cholesterol to CHD is that obtained from clinical trials in which cholesterol levels are lowered by dietary modifications or drugs. Several such trials have now been carried out, and the aggregate data strongly suggest that lowering cholesterol levels in hypercholesterolemic patients reduces the risk for CHD (Fig. 1.41). The decline in CHD risk within these studies is proportional to the reduction in cholesterol levels. Thus, not only does a high cholesterol level predispose to CHD, but a therapeutic reduction in cholesterol level reduces the risk of CHD.

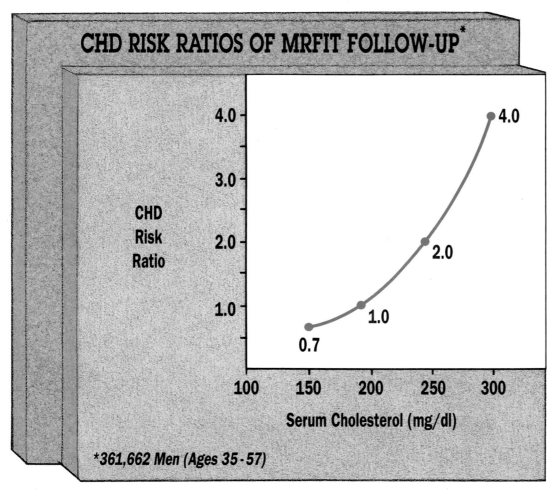

Fig. 1.42 CHD risk ratios for the MRFIT follow-up survey.

RISK RATIOS VS. ATTRIBUTABLE RISK

The relationship between cholesterol levels and CHD can be expressed not only in absolute terms but also in relative terms, or risk ratios. The latter is the ratio of absolute rates at two different cholesterol levels. Risk ratios for the MRFIT follow-up are shown in Figure 1.42. If we assign a ratio of 1.0 for a cholesterol level of 200 mg/dl, then for those whose average cholesterol is 250 mg/dl, the risk ratio is 2.0; and for a cholesterol level of 300 mg/dl, the ratio is 4.0. Thus, within the range of 200 to 250 mg/dl, for every 1.0 mg/dl rise in total cholesterol, the risk is increased by 1%. Because of the curvilinear nature of the curve, a 50 mg/dl reduction of cholesterol level below 200 mg/dl produces a fall in risk ratio of only 0.3, whereas a rise from 250 to 300 mg/dl enhances the risk ratio from 2.0 to 4.0.

The curve for the risk ratio is not the same at all ages. As the age increases, the increment in risk ratio declines for a given cholesterol level. This is illustrated for the data from the MRFIT study in Figure 1.43. These data might suggest that cholesterol plays a less important role in the causation of CHD in older people. However, the change in risk ratios does not take into account changes in absolute rates of CHD with aging. In other words, the absolute number of new cases of CHD that can be attributed to higher cholesterol is greater in older people than in younger people. Figure 1.44 shows the curves for this attributable risk at different ages in the MRFIT follow-up. Clearly, higher cholesterol levels do not lose their impact on CHD in older people; rather, if anything, the impact is enhanced.

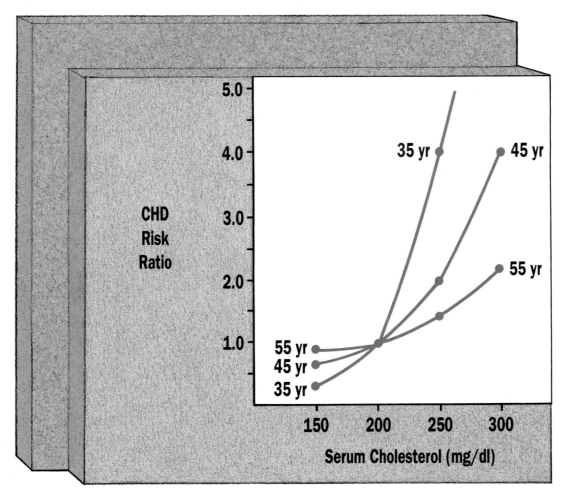

Fig. 1.43 CHD risk ratios for data from the MRFIT study showing decline in the increment in risk with increasing age.

CHOLESTEROL LEVELS AND TOTAL MORTALITY

The MRFIT data demonstrate a relation between cholesterol levels and CHD mortality. However, several epidemiologic studies suggest the occurrence of a J-shaped relation between cholesterol levels and total mortality. In other words, total mortality is highest at the highest cholesterol levels, but it also tends to rise with the lowest cholesterol concentrations. This finding could mean that low levels of cholesterol, as well as high, may be dangerous. One explanation for this finding may be that individuals with the lowest cholesterol levels at entry into a survey may already have a potentially fatal disease (e.g., early stage of cancer) or may be predisposed to a disease that will simultaneously lower the cholesterol level. In the absence of such a condition, a low cholesterol level may not be detrimental. Evidence to support this latter concept comes from the Framingham Heart Study. Those who had the lowest cholesterol levels at the time of first examination had the lowest *overall* mortality in the subsequent 30 years (Fig. 1.45). From these results, it appears that low cholesterol levels per se do not predispose to death, but rather the opposite.

LIPOPROTEIN FRACTIONS AND CHD RISK

LDL-Cholesterol and CHD Risk. Many investigators believe that LDL are the most atherogenic of all lipoproteins. LDL are relatively small, cholesterol-rich particles that can readily filter into the arterial wall. They also contain apo B-100, which should promote their entrapment in the arterial wall. Furthermore, LDL generally carry most of the cholesterol

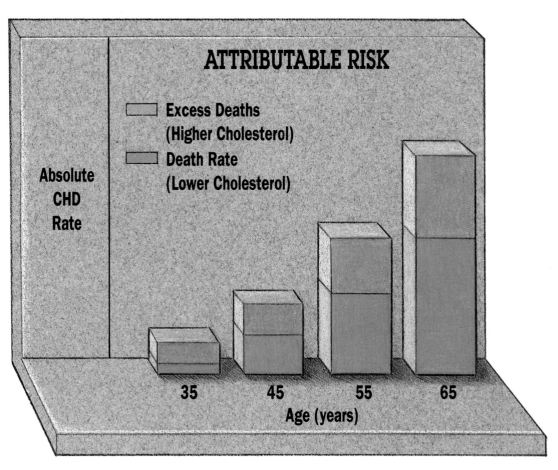

Fig. 1.44 Attributable risk of CHD at different ages in the MRFIT follow-up survey.

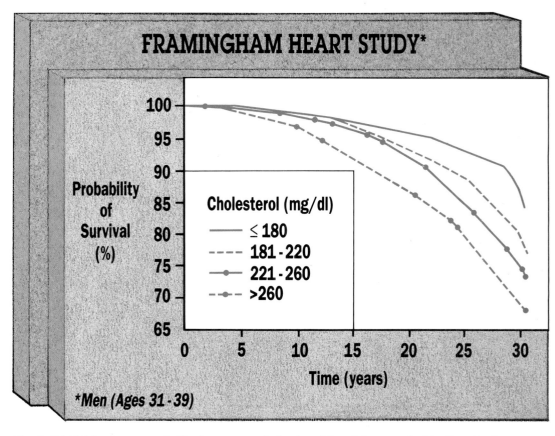

Fig. 1.45 Thirty-year mortality by serum cholesterol level for men in the Framingham Heart Study.

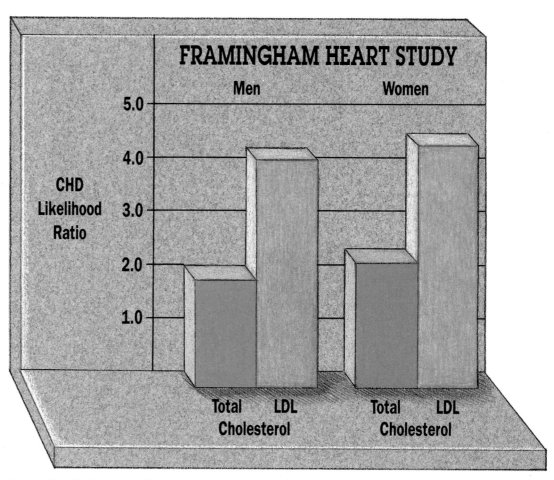

Fig. 1.46 Likelihood ratios for CHD of total cholesterol compared with LDL - cholesterol in men and women in the Framingham Heart Study.

in the serum. Indeed, the strong relation between total-cholesterol levels and CHD risk may exist because the measurement of total cholesterol is a good "surrogate" for LDL-cholesterol. In the Framingham Heart Study, the correlation was stronger between LDL-cholesterol levels and CHD risk than between total cholesterol and CHD risk; this is shown by the higher likelihood ratio for CHD of LDL-cholesterol compared with total cholesterol (Fig. 1.46). The higher the likelihood ratio, the greater is the strength of the correlation. This finding seems to support the notion that the LDL-cholesterol is a better predictor of CHD than the total cholesterol. If so, it provides a rationale for measurement of LDL-cholesterol for the purpose of making an accurate assessment of an individual's CHD risk or the efficacy of a particular cholesterol-lowering therapy.

VLDL-Cholesterol and CHD Risk. Evidence is mounting that cholesterol carried in VLDL also can be atherogenic. The dangerous form of VLDL-cholesterol may reside more with VLDL remnants than with newly secreted VLDL. Results of the Framingham Heart Study reveal

that VLDL-cholesterol levels (or their "surrogate," serum triglycerides) are significantly correlated with risk for CHD in both men and women. However, the relation between VLDL-cholesterol and CHD appears to be stronger in women than in men. As shown by likelihood ratios for CHD, VLDL-cholesterol in women emerged as being as strong an independent predictor of CHD as LDL-cholesterol, whereas for men its predictive power was less, being even less than that of total cholesterol (Fig. 1.47). The latter does not mean that VLDL-cholesterol is not atherogenic in men, but because of relatively low concentrations of VLDL-cholesterol in most individuals, it is not as good a predictor of CHD as total cholesterol. Recent evidence from the Framingham Heart Study shows that VLDL-cholesterol is still a significant predictor in men as well as in women, but it must be remembered that in most men only 15% to 20% of total cholesterol is carried in the VLDL fraction; thus, for most people, its total contribution to atherogenesis will be less than the contribution of LDL. In laboratory animals, a high level of VLDL-cholesterol almost certainly is atherogenic; in fact, for many species, the feeding of excess cholesterol results in an elevation of VLDL-cholesterol, not of LDL-cholesterol, and atherosclerosis develops rapidly.

Triglycerides and CHD Risk. Much dispute exists about the connection between triglyceride concentrations and the risk for CHD. Most epidemiologic studies reveal a positive correlation between triglyceride levels and the incidence of CHD by univariate analysis. However, triglycerides often lose their significance when multivariate analysis is carried out, that is, when other known risk factors are taken into account. Indeed, triglycerides per se probably are not atherogenic, and any connection between serum triglyceride levels and CHD probably can be explained by the presence of atherogenic, triglyceride-rich lipoproteins. For example, there is a high correlation between serum triglycerides and VLDL-cholesterol, and in general, the relationship between VLDL-cholesterol and CHD holds as well for triglycerides (see Fig. 1.47). Even so, the cholesterol in VLDL, not the triglyceride, most likely is the atherogenic component. These comments pertain primarily to the correlation between triglyceride levels and CHD rates in the general population. Many patients with clinical hypertriglyceridemia appear to be at increased risk for CHD, and this issue is considered in more detail in Unit 2.

IDL-Cholesterol and CHD Risk. In routine lipoprotein analysis, the IDL-cholesterol is not measured, but rather it is combined with LDL to produce an estimated "LDL-cholesterol." In several clinical investigations, however, IDL-cholesterol has emerged as an "independent" risk factor for CHD. This is important because it adds strength to the argument that LDL is not the exclusive atherogenic lipoprotein; and moreover, if IDL-cholesterol is atherogenic, then it is very likely that the other triglyceride-rich lipoprotein, VLDL, also has atherogenic potential.

HDL-Cholesterol and CHD Risk. Many epidemiologic investigations reveal a strong negative correlation between rates of CHD and the HDL-cholesterol level. For example, in the Framingham Heart study, a much stronger association was noted between HDL-cholesterol concentrations and CHD rates than for any other single lipid or lipoprotein fraction; this is shown by a comparison of likelihood ratios for CHD from that study (Fig. 1.48). HDL-cholesterol of all lipid fractions is the most highly correlated with CHD. Another way to view the relation between HDL-cholesterol levels

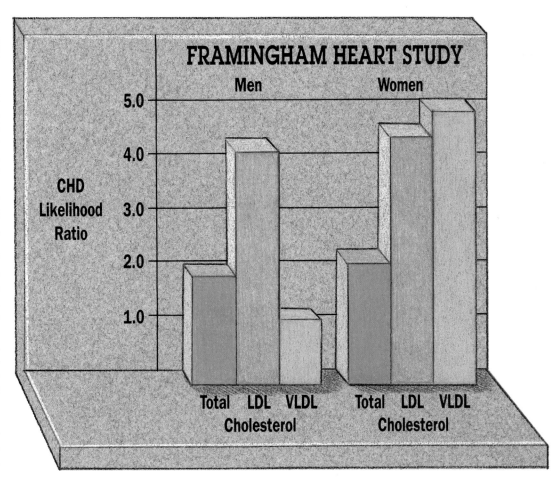

Fig. 1.47 Likelihood ratios for CHD of VLDL - cholesterol compared with total cholesterol and LDL - cholesterol in men and women in the Framingham Heart Study.

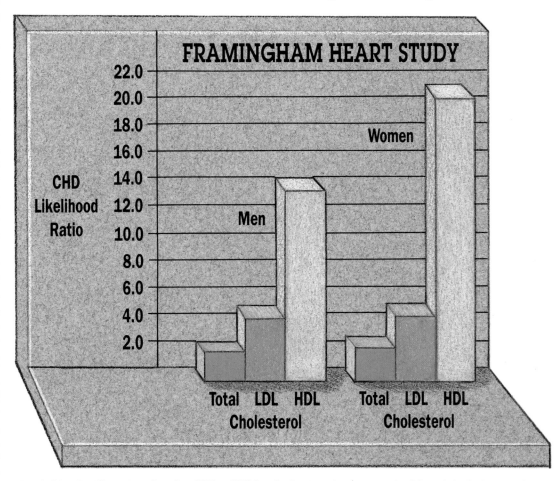

Fig. 1.48 Likelihood ratios for CHD of HDL - cholesterol compared with total cholesterol and LDL - cholesterol in men and women in the Framingham Heart Study.

Fig. 1.49 Risk ratios for CHD of total cholesterol and HDL-cholesterol. Data are those of the Framingham Heart Study.

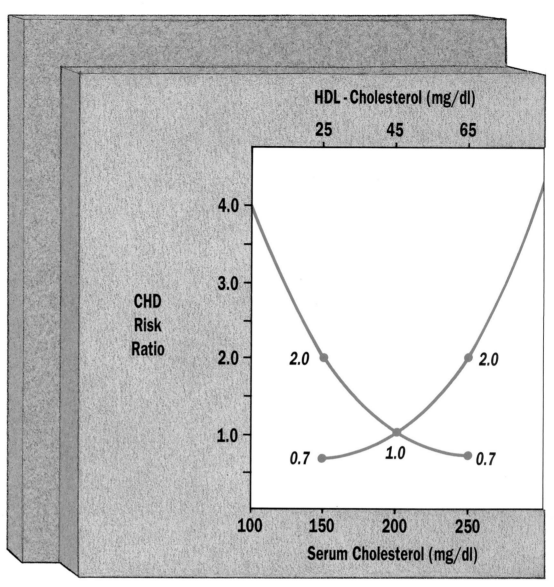

Fig. 1.50 Cholesterol ratios (LDL-C/HDL-C and TC/HDL-C) correlated with risk ratios for CHD in men in the Framingham Heart Study.

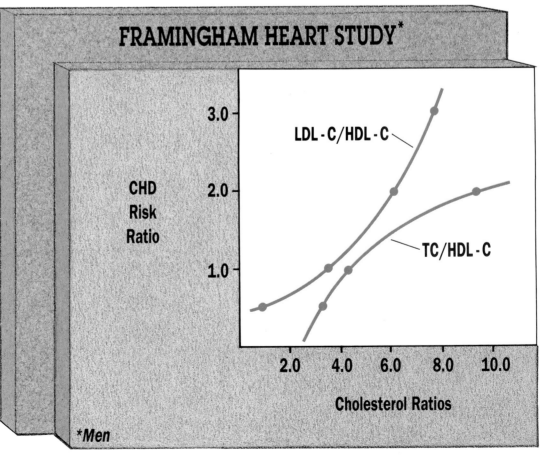

and CHD is shown in Figure 1.49, in which the data are again those from the Framingham Heart Study. Risk ratios for CHD are plotted simultaneously for total cholesterol and HDL-cholesterol. As indicated before, an increase in total cholesterol from 200 to 250 mg/dl essentially doubles the risk for CHD. On the other hand, reducing HDL-cholesterol levels from 45 to 25 mg/dl doubles the risk. Thus, for every 1.0 mg/dl increase in total cholesterol, the risk for CHD increases by about 1%, whereas for every 1.0 mg/dl decrease in HDL-cholesterol the risk of CHD rises by 2% to 3%.

Cholesterol Ratios and CHD Risk. Since the different cholesterol fractions are independently related to CHD risk, one way to simplify risk assessment is to compute ratios of lipid (or lipoprotein) fractions. Two frequently used ratios are the total cholesterol/HDL-cholesterol (TC/HDL-C) ratio and the LDL-cholesterol/HDL-cholesterol (LDL-C/HDL-C) ratio. In fact, in the Framingham Heart Study, the highest correlations with CHD among the lipid fractions are noted for these ratios. When Framingham data are used to compute CHD risk ratios against the TC/HDL-C ratio, a graph such as that shown in Figure 1.50 is obtained. If a TC/HDL-C ratio of 4.4 is assigned a CHD risk ratio of 1.0, a TC/HDL-C ratio of 3.4 cuts CHD risk in half, whereas a ratio of 9.6 doubles the risk. An even stronger correlation is noted for the LDL-C/HDL-C ratio. Although widely advocated, use of cholesterol ratios may be misleading, particularly at higher and lower levels of total cholesterol. For example, a high HDL-cholesterol level may not be protective in an individual with a marked increase in total (or LDL-) cholesterol, and a low HDL-cholesterol level may still be an important risk factor in individuals with relatively low concentrations of LDL-cholesterol.

OTHER CHD RISK FACTORS

Besides lipoproteins, several other risk factors contribute to the development of CHD. For the general population, the major risk factors are hypertension, smoking, and high serum cholesterol. As indicated previously, the serum total cholesterol is mainly a "surrogate" for LDL-cholesterol, but a high VLDL-cholesterol also is a risk factor. A low HDL-cholesterol deserves to be classified as a risk factor because of its correlation with a high incidence of CHD. Other significant risk factors are diabetes mellitus (hyperglycemia) and obesity. CHD risk ratios for hypertension (Fig. 1.51) and cigarette smoking (Fig. 1.52), derived

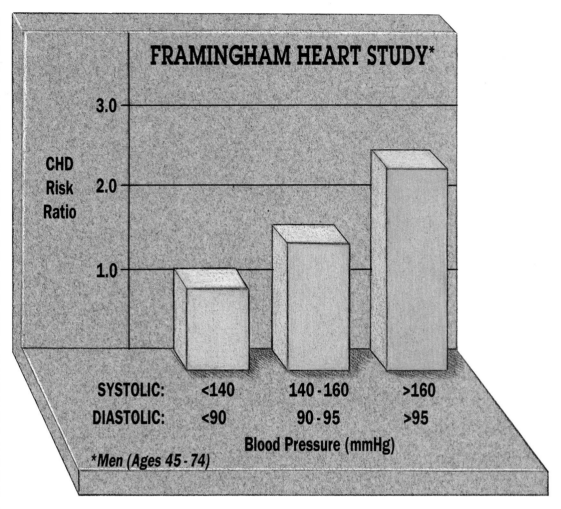

Fig. 1.51 Risk ratios for CHD correlated with hypertension in men in the Framingham Heart Study.

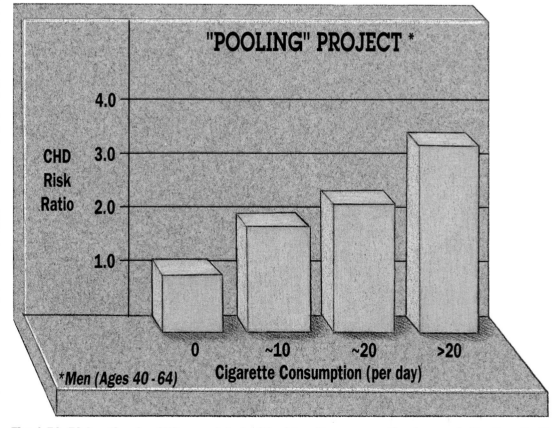

Fig. 1.52 Risk ratios for CHD correlated with cigarette consumption in men in the "pooling" project.

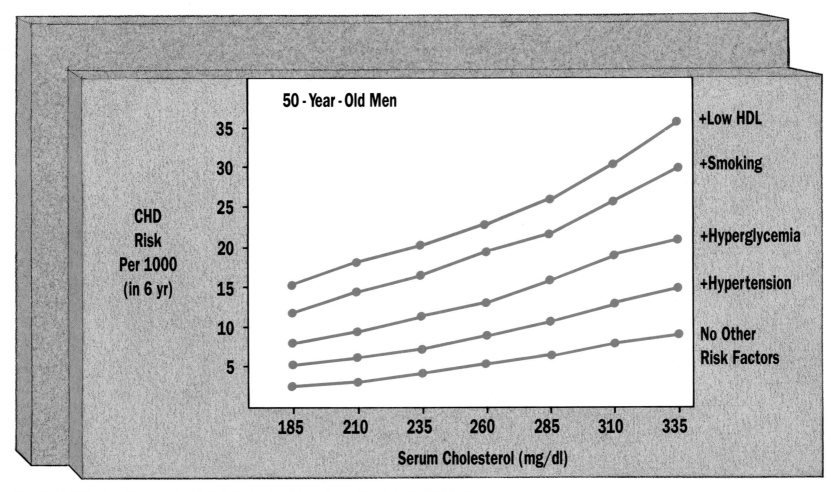

Fig. 1.53 Effects of increasing total cholesterol levels on the risk of CHD in the presence of other risk factors in men aged 50 years.

from large epidemiologic surveys, show a graded relationship between CHD risk and the rise of blood pressure or the intensity of smoking. The presence of diabetes mellitus essentially doubles the risk for CHD, whereas marked obesity enhances risk from one-and-one-half- to twofold. Recent data suggest that obesity is an "independent" risk factor for CHD; in other words, not only does it worsen other risk factors (i.e., hyperlipidemia, low HDL, hypertension, and diabetes), but it also raises the risk for CHD independently of these factors. The reason for the latter effect is unknown, but it may be related to the causation of left ventricular hypertrophy, a known cause of sudden coronary death.

INTERACTION OF RISK FACTORS

Not only do the risk factors act independently to increase the danger of myocardial infarction, but they also are additive with one another. This is illustrated in Figure 1.53, which shows the effects of increasing total cholesterol levels on the risk of CHD in the presence of other risk factors. With the inclusion of more risk factors, there is a progressive increase in coronary risk with increasing cholesterol levels. This observation provides a rationale for more vigorous treatment of hypercholesterolemia in patients with, rather than without, other coronary risk factors.

Unit Two

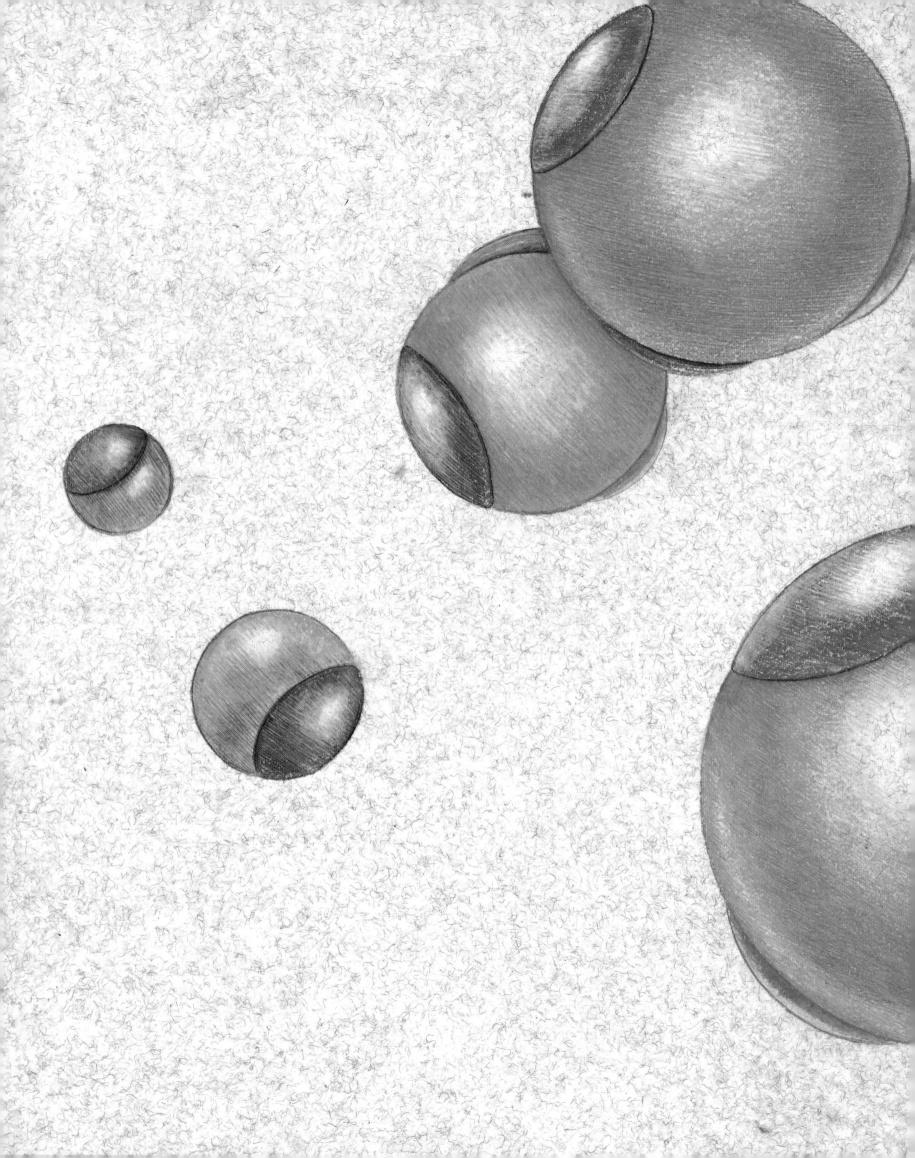

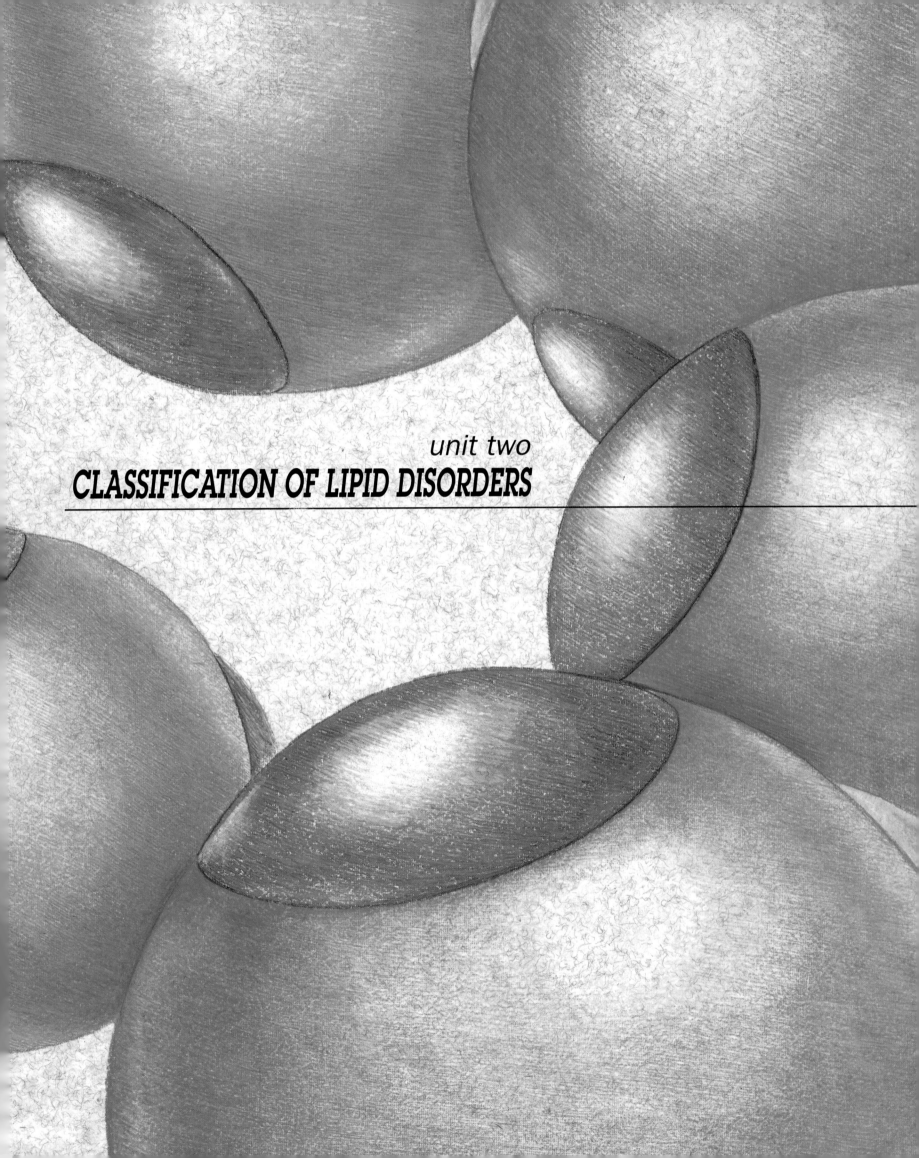

CLASSIFICATION OF LIPID DISORDERS

WHOM TO TEST?

Two approaches to the control of high serum cholesterol are the public health approach and the high-risk strategy. The public health approach attempts to modify the living habits of the general population–by changing the diet, by increasing exercise, and by reducing stress levels. This approach has been advocated by the American Heart Association over the past three decades. The high-risk strategy consists of finding people with high serum cholesterol (or other dyslipidemias) by testing individuals for serum cholesterol and other lipids. These approaches are complementary, and both will be required to obtain a maximal reduction of coronary heart disease (CHD) risk. Since the high-risk strategy requires the detection of patients with high blood cholesterol, an important question thus becomes: whom to test? (Fig. 2.1). Current recommendations are that the serum total cholesterol level should be measured on all adults over 20 years of age and on children of parents who have premature CHD or a history of dyslipidemia. It is not necessary to test all children and adolescents before age 20 years if they do not belong to high-risk families. Only the serum total cholesterol level need be measured. Subsequent measurements of triglycerides and/or lipoproteins should be made on the basis of the total cholesterol level and a judgment of an individual's overall risk status.

CLASSIFICATION OF BLOOD CHOLESTEROL

Three categories of serum cholesterol were defined by the adult treatment panel of the National Cholesterol Education Program (Fig. 2.2). A *desirable* level of serum cholesterol was defined as one measuring less than 200 mg/dl. Epidemiologic studies both within and between populations have shown that total cholesterol levels below 200 mg/dl have the lowest risk of CHD of all cholesterol categories. Even within the desirable range (i.e., below 200 mg/dl), the lowest values impart the least risk for CHD, but the rise in risk over this range is relatively small (see Unit 1).

Cholesterol readings within the range of 200 to 239 mg/dl are defined as *borderline-high* levels. Within this range, there is a progressive increase in risk, approximately doubling from 200 to 239 mg/dl. However, the absolute risk imparted by increasing cholesterol levels depends on the presence or absence of other risk factors (see Unit 1). For this reason, a borderline-high cholesterol level should induce greater concern in patients with CHD or other coronary risk factors than in those without CHD or other risk factors. This difference will affect the extent of workup of patients with borderline-high cholesterol levels, which will be described later in this section.

Cholesterol levels over 240 mg/dl are defined as *high* serum cholesterol. In

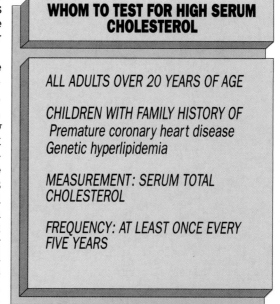

Fig. 2.1 Whom to test for high serum cholesterol.

Fig. 2.2 Categories of serum cholesterol as defined by the National Cholesterol Education Program.

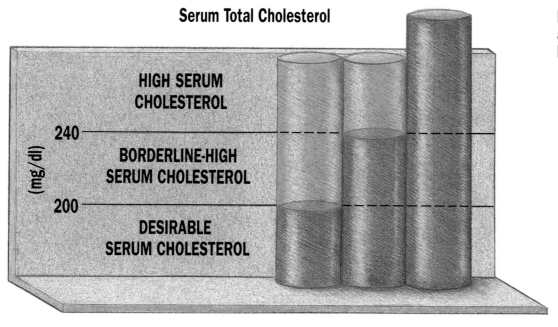

Serum Total Cholesterol

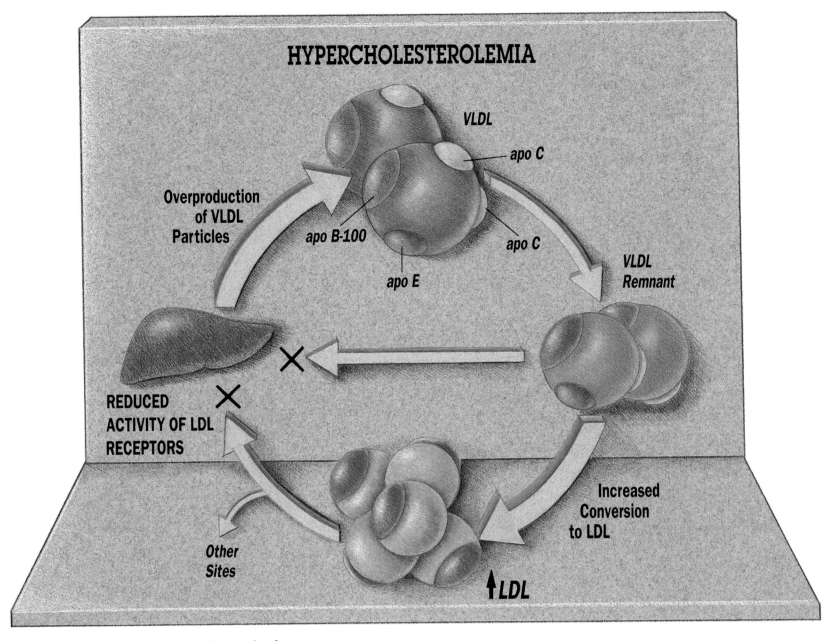

HYPERCHOLESTEROLEMIA

VLDL

apo C

Overproduction of VLDL Particles

apo B-100

apo E

apo C

VLDL Remnant

REDUCED ACTIVITY OF LDL RECEPTORS

Other Sites

Increased Conversion to LDL

↑LDL

Fig. 2.3 Mechanisms of hypercholesterolemia.

studies involving large populations, the risk for CHD with such cholesterol readings at least doubles, compared with levels less than 200 mg/dl. However, population data cannot be extended to all individuals; depending on the lipoprotein profile, the risk imparted by a given cholesterol level may be greater or less than the population average risk. Nonetheless, for any person, a level over 240 mg/dl requires further workup to better define the individual's relative risk.

CAUSES OF HYPERCHOLESTEROLEMIA

Four factors appear to contribute to the development of high serum cholesterol levels: (1) aging, (2) diet, (3) genetic predisposition, and (4) secondary causes. The common metabolic abnormalities in lipoprotein metabolism leading to high cholesterol levels are shown in Figure 2.3. For most people, an increase in total cholesterol concentrations is due to high levels of low-density

lipoprotein (LDL)-cholesterol. Two general mechanisms are responsible for increased LDL levels. The first is a decrease in LDL-receptor activity, leading to delayed clearance of both LDL and very low-density lipoprotein (VLDL) remnants. Moreover, the delay in clearance results in a greater conversion of VLDL remnants to LDL, which further raises LDL levels. The second abnormality is an overproduction of lipoproteins by the liver. An increased input of lipoproteins tends to

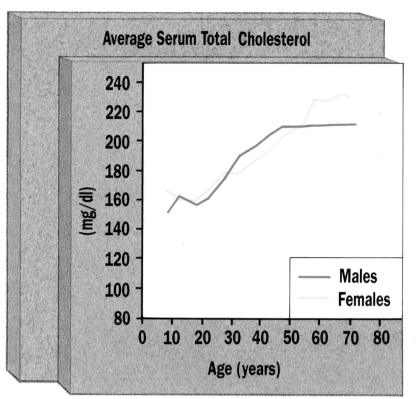

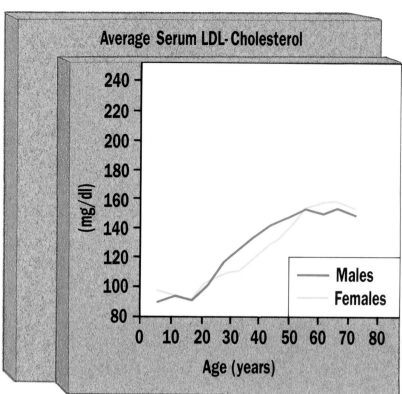

Fig. 2.4 Rises with age in (left) serum total cholesterol and (right) LDL-cholesterol.

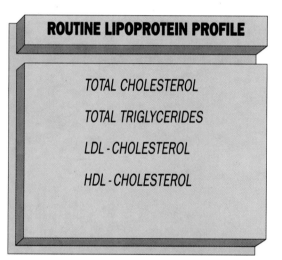

Fig. 2.5 Elements comprising the routine lipoprotein profile.

raise concentrations all along the lipoprotein cascade, i.e., VLDL, VLDL remnants, and LDL.

Levels of total cholesterol and LDL-cholesterol rise with age (Fig. 2.4). Mean levels of LDL-cholesterol increase by approximately 30 to 40 mg/dl from 20 years to 60 years of age. The cause of the rise of cholesterol levels with age is unknown. Our studies have shown that the two abnormalities responsible for hypercholesterolemia–increased production of lipoproteins and decreased clearance of LDL-cholesterol–contribute to the rise of LDL with increasing age. Multiple metabolic changes, among them, a decrease in metabolic rate, increasing body weight, changing body composition, and the long-term effect of a hypercholesterolemic diet, are probably responsible for the rise of cholesterol levels with age.

All the other causes of hypercholesterolemia, such as diet, genetics, and other diseases, generally induce hypercholesterolemia by the mechanisms outlined in Figure 2.3. The effects of inherited metabolic diseases and secondary causes are examined in the sections that follow; the influence of diet is discussed in Unit 3.

LIPOPROTEIN PROFILE
LIPID COMPONENTS

The routine lipoprotein profile consists of measurement of serum total cholesterol, total triglycerides, LDL-cholesterol, and high-density lipoprotein (HDL)-cholesterol (Fig 2.5). The total cholesterol and triglyceride levels can be determined directly on fasting serum. HDL-cholesterol is determined on the supranatant after precipitation of apolipoprotein-B-containing lipoproteins (VLDL and LDL). LDL-cholesterol is calculated indirectly by the equation: LDL-cholesterol = [total cholesterol] – [triglyceride/5] – [HDL-cholesterol]. This equation holds for triglyceride levels up to, but not above 400 mg/dl. If an accurate LDL-cholesterol value is required for markedly hypertriglyceridemic serum, the specimen must be subjected to ultracentrifugation to remove the excess triglyceride.

INDICATIONS FOR LIPOPROTEIN PROFILE

The lipoprotein profile (Fig. 2.6) should be obtained for patients with a high serum cholesterol (greater than 240

INDICATIONS FOR LIPOPROTEIN PROFILE

SERUM TOTAL CHOLESTEROL OVER 240 MG/DL

SERUM TOTAL CHOLESTEROL IN THE RANGE OF 200 TO 239 MG/DL
+ Coronary heart disease (CHD)
or
+ Two other CHD risk factors *

* One of these risk factors may be the male sex. See also Figure 2.7.

Fig. 2.6   Indications for obtaining a lipoprotein profile.

RISK FACTORS FOR CORONARY HEART DISEASE (CHD)

MALE SEX

FAMILY HISTORY OF PREMATURE CHD

CIGARETTE SMOKING

HYPERTENSION

LOW HDL-CHOLESTEROL (< 35 MG/DL)

DIABETES MELLITUS

HISTORY OF CEREBRAL OR PERIPHERAL VASCULAR DISEASE

Fig. 2.7   Risk factors for coronary heart disease.

Fig. 2.8   Categories of serum LDL-cholesterol.

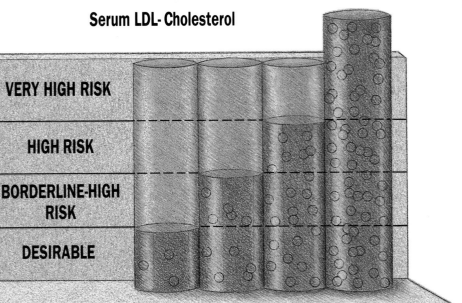

Serum LDL- Cholesterol

VERY HIGH RISK

190

HIGH RISK

160

BORDERLINE-HIGH RISK

130

DESIRABLE

(mg/dl)

mg/dl) or patients otherwise deemed to be at high risk on the basis of having definite CHD (i.e., a history of myocardial infarction or angina pectoris) or two other CHD risk factors (Fig. 2.7). The measurement of lipoproteins in patients with borderline-high cholesterol (200 to 239 mg/dl) is optional if patients are free of CHD or two other CHD risk factors; many authorities advocate obtaining a lipoprotein profile

for the latter patients, especially for younger men if not for all others.

CLASSIFICATION OF LDL-CHOLESTEROL

Levels of serum LDL-cholesterol less than 130 mg/dl are called *desirable* and those between 130 and 159 mg/dl are termed *borderline-high risk* (Fig. 2.8). The *high-risk* category of LDL-cholesterol is marked by readings

between 160 and 190 mg/dl and the *very high-risk* category by levels above 190 mg/dl. Classification by LDL-cholesterol should be used in assessing a patient's lipid risk status in preference to measurement of serum total cholesterol alone. Although there is a high correlation between total cholesterol and LDL-cholesterol levels in large populations, this correlation does not necessarily hold for individuals;

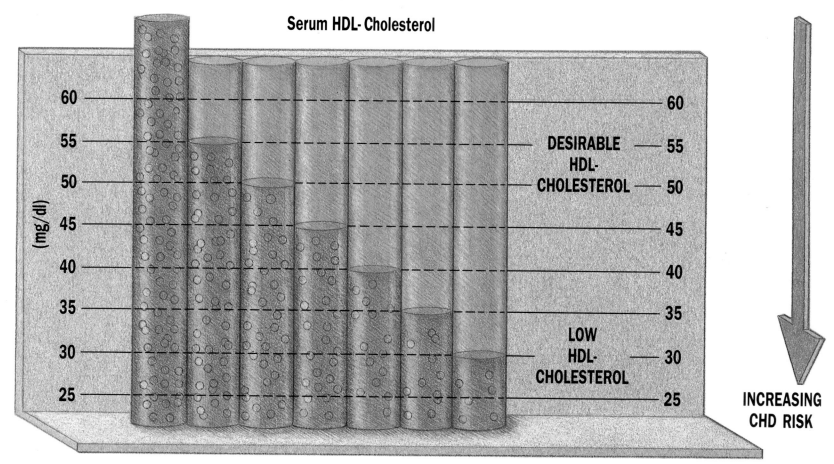

Serum HDL-Cholesterol

DESIRABLE
HDL-
CHOLESTEROL

LOW
HDL-
CHOLESTEROL

INCREASING
CHD RISK

Fig. 2.9 Categories of serum HDL-cholesterol and their relation to increasing risk of coronary heart disease (CHD).

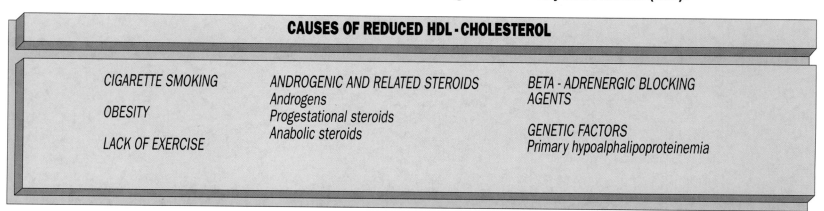

CAUSES OF REDUCED HDL - CHOLESTEROL

CIGARETTE SMOKING

OBESITY

LACK OF EXERCISE

ANDROGENIC AND RELATED STEROIDS
Androgens
Progestational steroids
Anabolic steroids

BETA - ADRENERGIC BLOCKING
AGENTS

GENETIC FACTORS
Primary hypoalphalipoproteinemia

Fig. 2.10 Causes of reduced serum HDL-cholesterol.

consequently, a lipoprotein profile is required to fully assess a patient's risk.

HYPOALPHALIPOPROTEINEMIA

An HDL-cholesterol level below 35 mg/dl is defined as *abnormal* or *"low."* However, as shown in Figure 2.9, the risk for CHD increases as HDL-cholesterol levels fall. CHD risk is distinctly increased at a level below 35 mg/dl, and this value can be used for setting goals of therapy for hypercholesterolemia.

A reduced level of HDL-cholesterol may result from several causes (Fig. 2.10). These include cigarette smoking, obesity, lack of exercise, andro-

genic and related steroids, beta-adrenergic blocking agents, and genetic factors.

Patients with genetic (primary) hypoalphalipoproteinemia often have HDL-cholesterol levels in the range of 20 to 29 mg/dl. The metabolic abnormalities responsible for such low concentrations of HDL-cholesterol are unknown, but they may be related to abnormalities in metabolism of the apolipoproteins (apo) A-I and A-II. Most of the secondary causes of low HDL-cholesterol generally do not produce such a severe depression in HDL levels; more commonly, they reduce HDL-cholesterol to the range of 30 to 39 mg/dl. An exception is anabolic

steroids, which, taken in large doses, can reduce HDL levels to 15 to 25 mg/dl.

HYPERTRIGLYCERIDEMIA
CLASSIFICATION OF SERUM TRIGLYCERIDES

A serum triglyceride level below 250 mg/dl is called *desirable.* Measurements in the range of 250 to 500 mg/dl can be designated *moderate,* or *"borderline,"* hypertriglyceridemia. Above 500 mg/dl, *marked* (*definite*) hypertriglyceridemia exists (Fig. 2.11). When triglyceride levels exceed 500 mg/dl, the serum usually contains chylomicrons in addition to VLDL; and at concentrations above

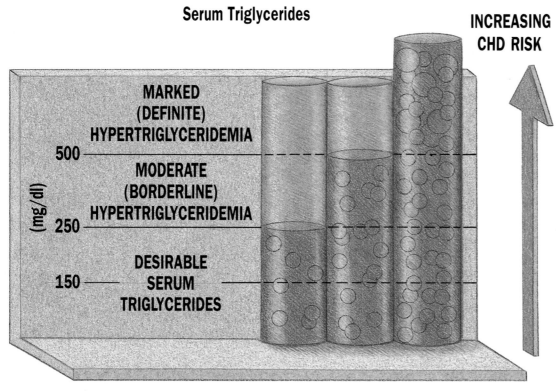

Serum Triglycerides

INCREASING CHD RISK

MARKED
(DEFINITE)
HYPERTRIGLYCERIDEMIA

500

MODERATE
(BORDERLINE)
HYPERTRIGLYCERIDEMIA

(mg/dl)

250

DESIRABLE
SERUM
TRIGLYCERIDES

150

Fig. 2.11 Categories of serum triglyceride levels and their relation to increasing risk of coronary heart disease (CHD).

1,000 mg/dl, chylomicrons typically predominate. Several studies have shown a positive correlation between triglyceride levels and the risk for CHD. This relationship has been noted even across the so-called normal range of serum triglycerides. However, when all the data are evaluated, it appears that elevated triglycerides per se are not a risk factor for CHD. Although many patients with hypertriglyceridemia develop premature CHD, this occurrence appears to be related to defects in lipoprotein metabolism that accompany high triglyceride levels.

METABOLIC CONSEQUENCES OF HYPERTRIGLYCERIDEMIA

The most common lipoprotein abnormalities produced by hypertriglyceridemia are increased concentrations of chylomicron remnants, VLDL remnants, and intermediate-density lipoprotein (IDL); as well as decreased levels of HDL-cholesterol, and the presence of small, dense LDL particles (Fig. 2.12). These abnormalities apparently result from both metabolic alterations and physicochemical changes secondary to the hypertriglyceridemic

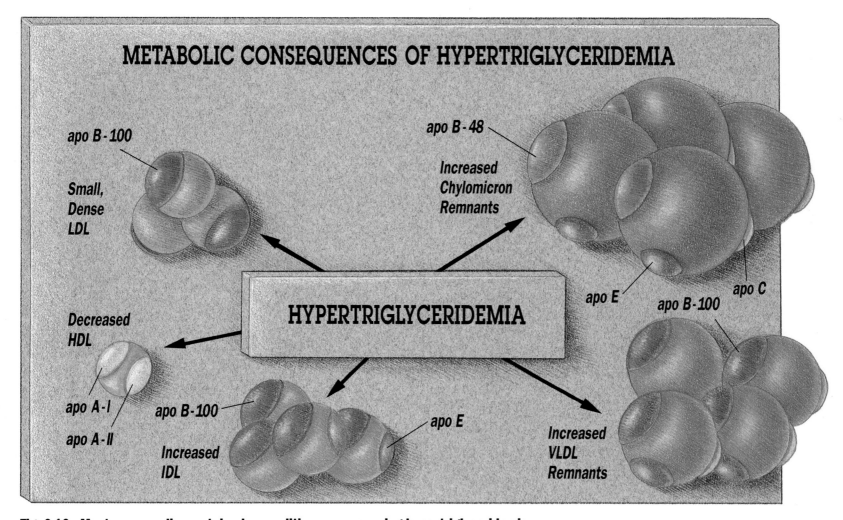

METABOLIC CONSEQUENCES OF HYPERTRIGLYCERIDEMIA

apo B-100

Small,
Dense
LDL

apo B-48

Increased
Chylomicron
Remnants

HYPERTRIGLYCERIDEMIA

apo E

apo B-100

apo C

Decreased
HDL

apo A-I

apo A-II

apo B-100

Increased
IDL

apo E

Increased
VLDL
Remnants

Fig. 2.12 Most common lipoprotein abnormalities accompanying hypertriglyceridemia.

Fig. 2.13   Causes of hypertriglyceridemia.

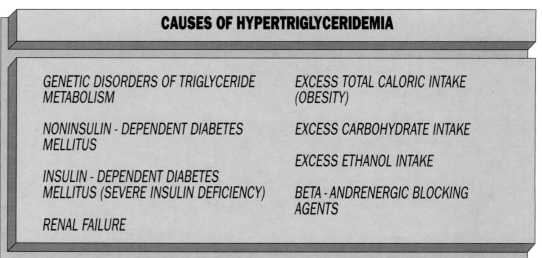

CAUSES OF HYPERTRIGLYCERIDEMIA

GENETIC DISORDERS OF TRIGLYCERIDE METABOLISM	*EXCESS TOTAL CALORIC INTAKE (OBESITY)*
NONINSULIN - DEPENDENT DIABETES MELLITUS	*EXCESS CARBOHYDRATE INTAKE*
INSULIN - DEPENDENT DIABETES MELLITUS (SEVERE INSULIN DEFICIENCY)	*EXCESS ETHANOL INTAKE*
RENAL FAILURE	*BETA - ADRENERGIC BLOCKING AGENTS*

Fig. 2.14   Complex interaction of primary, secondary, and dietary factors contributing to mixed hyperlipidemia.

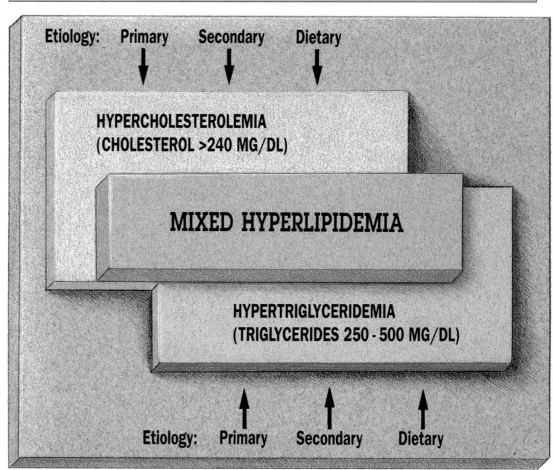

state. All of them have been implicated in atherogenesis. Thus, whereas elevated triglyceride levels per se may not be directly atherogenic, the metabolic consequences of hypertriglyceridemia appear to increase the risk for CHD.

CAUSES OF HYPERTRIGLYCERIDEMIA

Elevated levels of plasma triglycerides can have multiple causes (Fig. 2.13). Several different genetic abnormalities in triglyceride metabolism have been identified. These abnormalities produce a spectrum of increases in serum triglycerides, which ranges from high normal to moderate to severe. Hypertriglyceridemia can be secondary to other diseases, such as diabetes mellitus and renal failure, or to excessive intake of total calories (obesity), carbohydrates, and ethanol. Finally, concomitant drug use, notably beta-adrenergic blocking agents, can raise serum triglyceride levels.

MIXED HYPERLIPIDEMIA

Many patients have elevations of both cholesterol and triglyceride levels. Serum total cholesterol exceeding 240 mg/dl and a triglyceride level in the range of 250 to 500 mg/dl can be called mixed hyperlipidemia. Multiple factors (primary, secondary, and dietary) often contribute to these elevations. As shown in Figure 2.14, there can be a complex interaction among the various causes, and it is not unusual

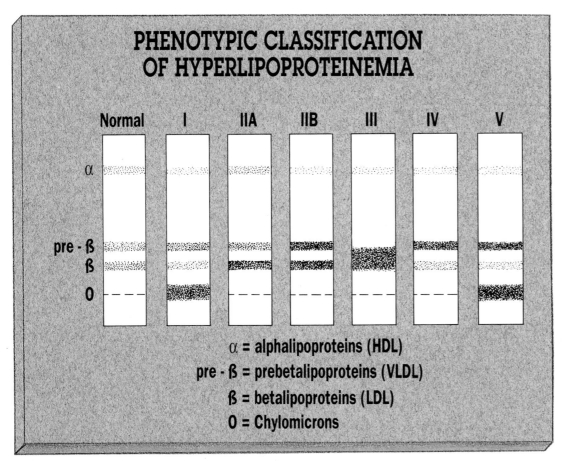

PHENOTYPIC CLASSIFICATION OF HYPERLIPOPROTEINEMIA

Normal   I   IIA   IIB   III   IV   V

α

pre - ß

ß

0

α = alphalipoproteins (HDL)

pre - ß = prebetalipoproteins (VLDL)

ß = betalipoproteins (LDL)

0 = Chylomicrons

Fig. 2.15 (Top) Phenotypic classification of hyperlipoproteinemia (HLP) based on patterns observed on paper electrophoresis. (Bottom) Types of HLP defined by increases in lipoprotein fractions.

TYPES OF HLP DEFINED BY INCREASES IN LIPOPROTEIN FRACTIONS

TYPE	INCREASED LIPOPROTEIN FRACTION(S)
I	Chylomicrons
IIA	· LDL
IIB	LDL and VLDL
III	beta-VLDL
IV	VLDL
V	VLDL and chylomicrons

to have more than two causative factors in a single patient. Most patients with mixed hyperlipidemia are at increased risk for CHD, and this appears to be a result both of elevated cholesterol levels and the metabolic consequences of hypertriglyceridemia.

HYPERLIPOPROTEINEMIA (HLP)
PHENOTYPIC CLASSIFICATION OF HLP

The phenotypic classification of HLP was originally based on the pattern of lipoproteins observed on paper electrophoresis (Fig. 2.15, top). In this system, betalipoproteins correspond to LDL, prebetalipoproteins to VLDL, broad betalipoproteins to beta-VLDL, alphalipoproteins to HDL, and the origin (no migration) to chylomicrons. According to this classification, six patterns of HLP were defined by increases in one or two lipoprotein fractions (Fig. 2.15, bottom). This classification still has conceptual utility, although paper electrolysis is rarely employed at present. Several of the phenotypes can be inferred from

values obtained from the lipoprotein profile, although more detailed studies are required for the definite identification of types I and III HLP.

SERUM PATTERNS OF HLP

Visual inspection of the serum after it has been allowed to sit overnight in the refrigerator often provides valuable information about the type of lipoprotein abnormality present. The various patterns can be compared with the normal straw color of serum having no

SERUM PATTERNS OF HYPERLIPOPROTEINEMIA

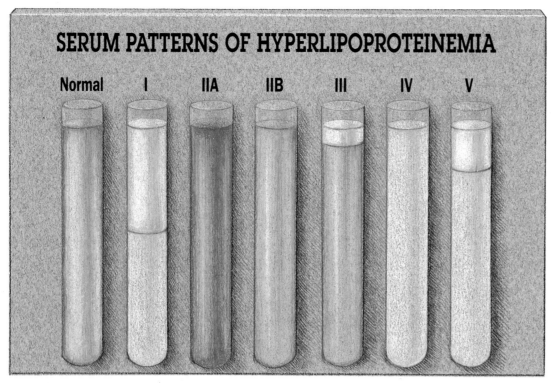

Normal   I   IIA   IIB   III   IV   V

Fig. 2.16 Serum patterns of hyperlipoproteinemia.

turbidity (Fig. 2.16). Type I HLP is indicated by a large creamy layer of chylomicrons that occupies the upper half of the tube; the lower half often has a faint turbidity. In type IIA, the serum is not turbid but has a deeper orange color due to increased quantities of carotene-carrying LDL. In type IIB, the same deep-orange color is combined with moderate turbidity throughout the tube due to an increase of LDL and VLDL. The serum of type III HLP has a similar appearance except for the frequent presence of a small quantity of chylomicrons at the top of the tube. In type IV HLP, the serum is turbid throughout, and in type V a "creaming" layer of chylomicrons is added to the turbidity of the whole tube.

TYPE I HLP

Type I HLP is characterized by severe chylomicronemia, which is secondary to a congenital deficiency of either lipoprotein lipase or apo C-II, the apoprotein required to activate lipoprotein lipase

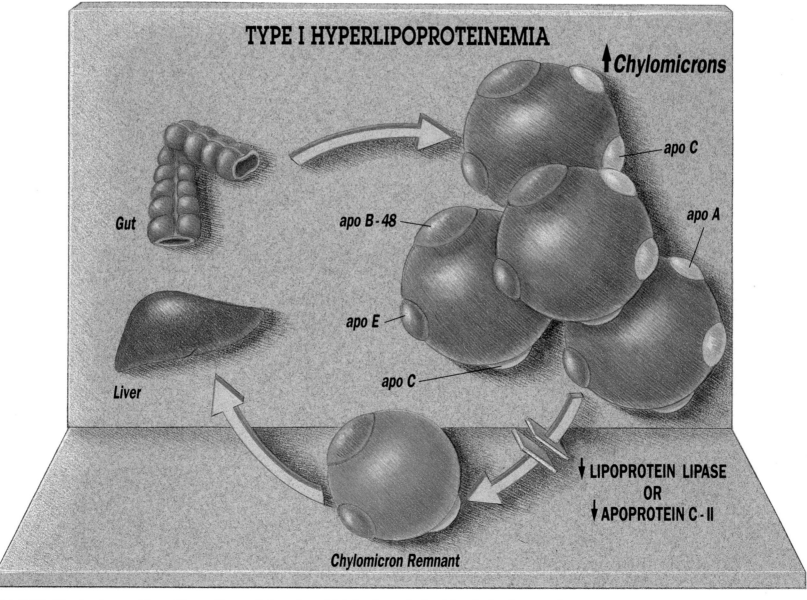

Fig. 2.17 Mechanisms of type I hyperlipoproteinemia, which is characterized by chylomicronemia.

(Fig. 2.17) Chylomicronemia is worsened by a high-fat diet, in which case triglyceride levels can range from 2,000 to 5,000 mg/dl. When levels reach these heights, patients are in danger of developing various complications (Fig. 2.18), foremost among them, acute pancreatitis. They may also manifest eruptive skin xanthomas and lipemia retinalis. Although type I HLP is a rare condition, its diagnosis is important to save the patient from repeated attacks of acute pancreatitis. The condition usually becomes manifest in early infancy or childhood.

TYPE II HLP

This phenotype represents an increase in LDL. In the past, the term type II was reserved for very high levels of LDL-cholesterol (i.e., over 190 mg/dl). The type II phenotype can be produced by either genetic abnormalities or other disease (these are discussed later in this unit). Type IIA refers to an increase in lipoproteins restricted to LDL, whereas, type IIB is marked by increases in LDL and VLDL.

TYPE III HLP

Type III HLP, also called familial dysbetalipoproteinemia, is characterized by an accumulation of beta-VLDL in the serum (Fig. 2.19). The necessary genetic defect for this condition is the homozygous state for apo E-2. Since apo E-2 has a low affinity for LDL receptors, its presence on VLDL particles imparts a defective clearance of VLDL remnants. Because of their delayed clearance, VLDL remnants acquire increased amounts of cholesterol esters and thereby are converted into beta-VLDL. Many individuals who have the E-2/E-2 genotype, however, have only mild accumulation of VLDL

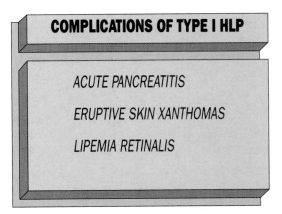

COMPLICATIONS OF TYPE I HLP

ACUTE PANCREATITIS

ERUPTIVE SKIN XANTHOMAS

LIPEMIA RETINALIS

Fig. 2.18 Complications of type I hyperlipoproteinemia.

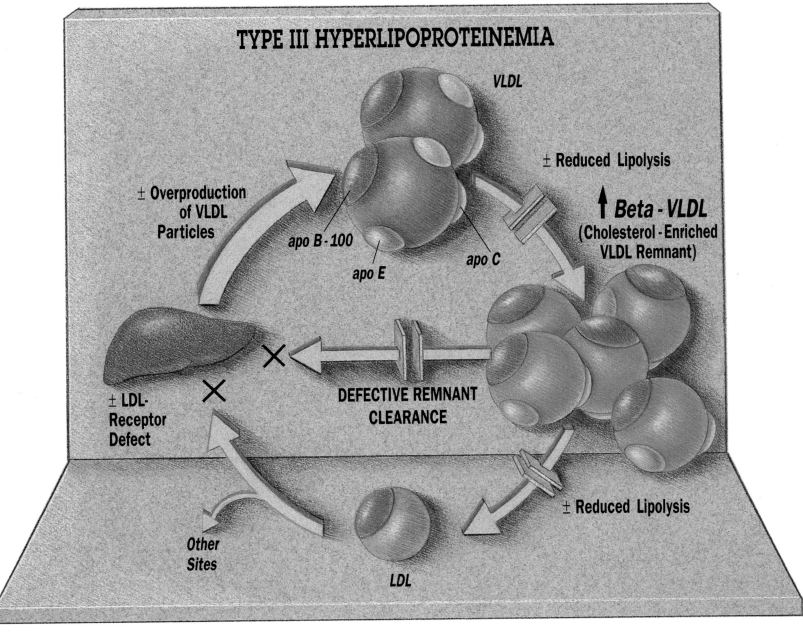

Fig. 2.19 Mechanisms of type III hyperlipoproteinemia, which exhibits an increased fraction of beta-VLDL.

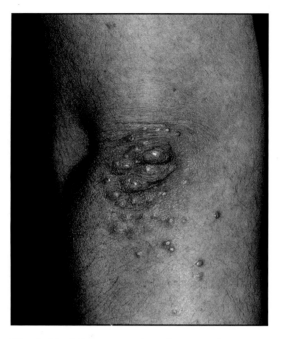

Fig. 2.20 Tuberous and tuberoeruptive xanthomas of the elbow secondary to type III hyperlipoproteinemia. (Courtesy of Jean Davignon, MD, Montreal, Quebec, Canada)

remnants and do not develop frank type III HLP. Consequently, it is postulated that concomitant defects in lipoprotein metabolism must be present for serum lipid levels to reach abnormal heights. Concomitant defects may be overproduction of VLDL, defective lypolysis of VLDL-triglycerides, or reduced activity of LDL receptors.

The diagnosis of type III HLP should be suggested by approximately equal elevations of serum cholesterol and triglycerides. A presumptive diagnosis can be made by finding broad betalipoprotein on electrophoresis or a high ratio of cholesterol to triglycerides (> 0.3) in VLDL. A definitive diagnosis depends on the finding of the E-2/E-2 pattern of apo E on isoelectric focusing or by genetic testing. Patients with type III HLP are prone to develop tuberous xanthomas (Fig. 2.20) and premature CHD.

TYPE IV HLP

This phenotype refers to an increase in VLDL levels. Triglyceride concentrations generally are in the range of 250 to 500 mg/dl, although they may be somewhat higher. Causes of type IV HLP are multiple–genetic, other diseases, or dietary. The first two of these causes are considered in this unit; dietary causes are discussed in Unit 3.

TYPE V HLP

This phenotype is recognized by high levels of both VLDL and chylomicrons (Fig. 2.21). Patients with this disorder usually have a dual defect in lipoprotein metabolism. Like patients with type I HLP, they have defective lipolysis of triglyceride-rich lipoproteins, although the lipolytic defect is less severe. Lipoprotein-lipase levels may be reduced, but they are not absent. A second defect in triglyceride metabolism is an overproduction of VLDL-triglycerides. The latter can occur on a genetic basis or secondary to diabetes mellitus, obesity, or excess alcohol intake. Type V HLP frequently does not become manifest until adulthood. When

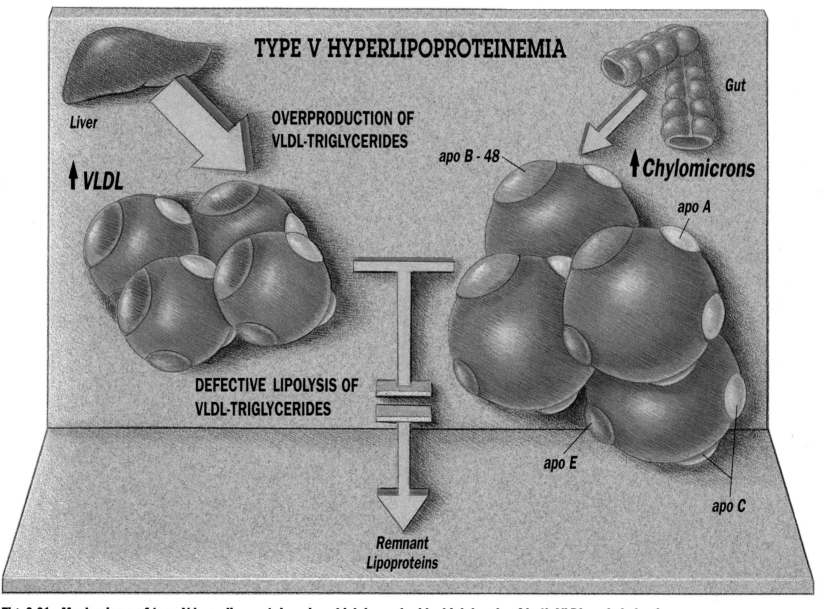

Fig. 2.21   Mechanisms of type V hyperlipoproteinemia, which is marked by high levels of both VLDL and chylomicrons.

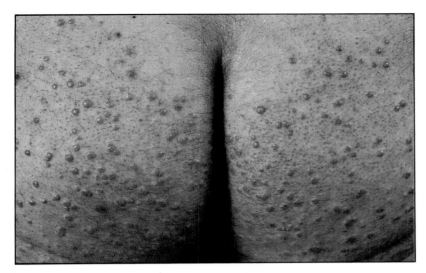

Fig. 2.22 Eruptive skin xanthomas of the buttocks secondary to type V hyperlipoproteinemia. (Courtesy of Jean Davignon, MD, Montreal, Quebec, Canada)

COMMON GENETIC HYPERLIPIDEMIAS

FAMILIAL HYPERCHOLESTEROLEMIA

POLYGENIC HYPERCHOLESTEROLEMIA

FAMILIAL DEFECTIVE APOLIPOPROTEIN B-100

FAMILIAL HYPERTRIGLYCERIDEMIA

FAMILIAL COMBINED HYPERLIPIDEMIA

Fig. 2.23 Common genetic hyperlipidemias.

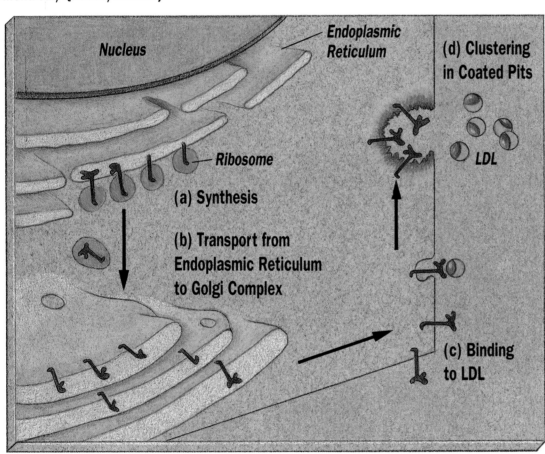

Fig. 2.24 Genetic defects underlying familial hypercholesterolemia: abnormalities in (a) LDL-receptor synthesis in the endoplasmic reticulum, (b) the transport of receptors to the Golgi complex, (c) the binding of receptors to LDL, and (d) the clustering of receptors in coated pits.

chylomicronemia becomes severe, patients also may develop eruptive skin xanthomas (Fig. 2.22), which are often harbingers of acute pancreatitis.

COMMON GENETIC HYPERLIPIDEMIAS

The evaluation of a patient with high serum cholesterol or other dyslipidemia requires consideration of the presence of an inherited metabolic defect. Because of the complexity of the lipoprotein system, inherited defects at multiple sites of metabolism are relatively common. Some of the more prevalent forms of genetic hyperlipidemias are presented

in Figure 2.23. These include familial hypercholesterolemia, polygenic hypercholesterolemia, the recently described familial defective apo B-100, familial hypertriglyceridemia, and familial combined hyperlipidemia. Each of these abnormalities is considered separately in the text that follows.

FAMILIAL HYPERCHOLESTEROLEMIA (FH)

The defect underlying FH is a genetic deficiency of LDL-receptor activity. The inheritance of two normal genes encoding the synthesis of LDL receptors –one from the father and one from the mother– is required to maintain a de-

sirable level of LDL-cholesterol. In one in 500 people, one gene is defective, and consequently, the affected person has only half the normal number of LDL receptors. As a result, the LDL-cholesterol levels are raised to twice the normal values. This condition is called *heterozygous* FH. Rarely, in one in 1,000,000 people, abnormal genes for the LDL receptor are inherited from both parents, producing *homozygous* FH. In this case, the affected patient has cholesterol levels in the range of 700 to 1,000 mg/dl. Multiple genetic defects in synthesis or expression of LDL receptors have been identified (Fig. 2.24). Abnormalities have been recognized in

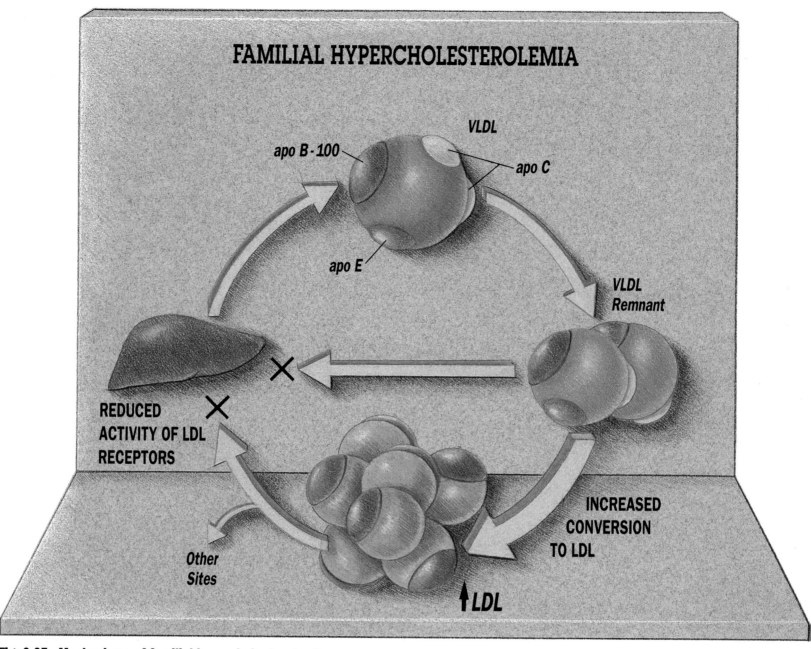

FAMILIAL HYPERCHOLESTEROLEMIA

apo B - 100

VLDL

apo C

apo E

VLDL Remnant

REDUCED ACTIVITY OF LDL RECEPTORS

Other Sites

INCREASED CONVERSION TO LDL

↑LDL

Fig. 2.25 Mechanisms of familial hypercholesterolemia.

the synthesis of LDL receptors in the endoplasmic reticulum, in the transport of newly synthesized receptors to the Golgi complex, in the binding of receptors to LDL, and in their clustering in coated pits. All of these defects produce the same clinical picture: severe hypercholesterolemia. The mechanisms of FH are those outlined in Figure 2.25, namely, retarded clearance of LDL and VLDL remnants and an increased conversion of VLDL to LDL.

Patients with heterozygous FH are prone to premature CHD. Affected men

often have myocardial infarction in their fourth or fifth decade, whereas in women the risk of myocardial infarction increases markedly after menopause. An important clinical sign is tendon xanthomas, which usually occur on the extensor tendons of the hands and the Achilles tendons (Fig. 2.26). Corneal arcus is another common finding. Since the defect is inherited as a monogenic-dominant disorder (Fig. 2.27), family screening usually reveals FH in half of first-degree relatives.

POLYGENIC HYPERCHOLESTEROLEMIA

Most patients with moderate-to-severe hypercholesterolemia do not have overt heterozygous FH. In most instances, however, genetic factors probably contribute to elevated LDL-cholesterol levels. Since LDL levels in polygenic hypercholesterolemia are rarely as high as in heterozygous FH, the genetic defects must impart less severe changes in LDL metabolism. The nature of these defects is not well understood for most patients; however, in recent years several spe-

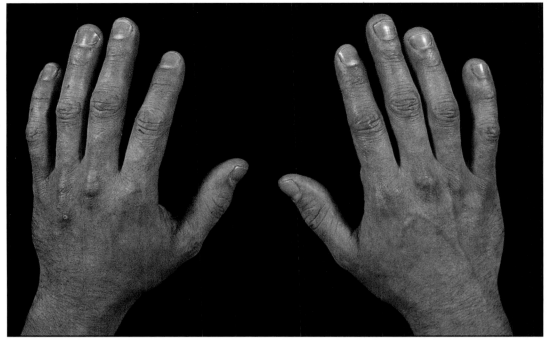
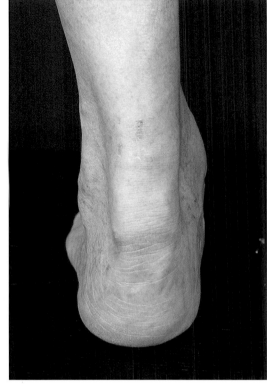

Fig. 2.26 (Left, right) Tendon xanthomas secondary to familial hypercholesterolemia. (Courtesy of Jean Davignon, MD, Montreal, Quebec, Canada)

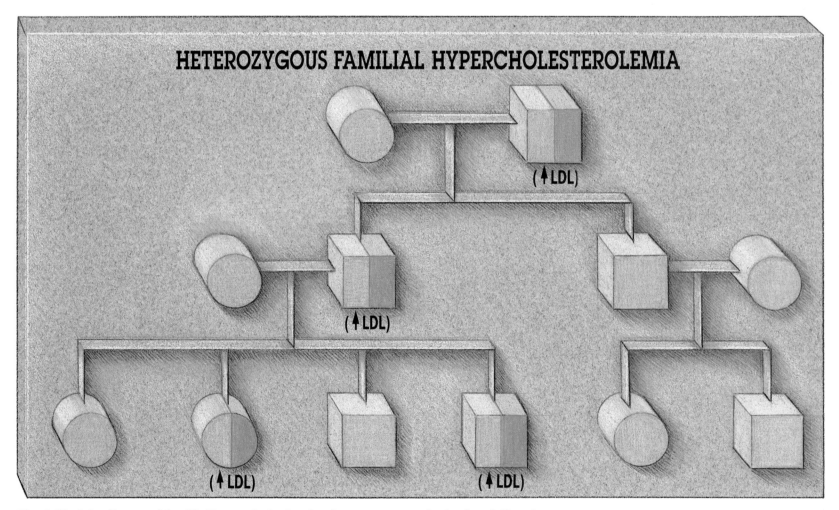

HETEROZYGOUS FAMILIAL HYPERCHOLESTEROLEMIA

(↑LDL)

(↑LDL)

(↑LDL)

(↑LDL)

Fig. 2.27 Inheritance of familial hypercholesterolemia as a monogenic-dominant disorder.

Fig. 2.28 Metabolic abnormalities responsible for polygenic hypercholesterolemia.

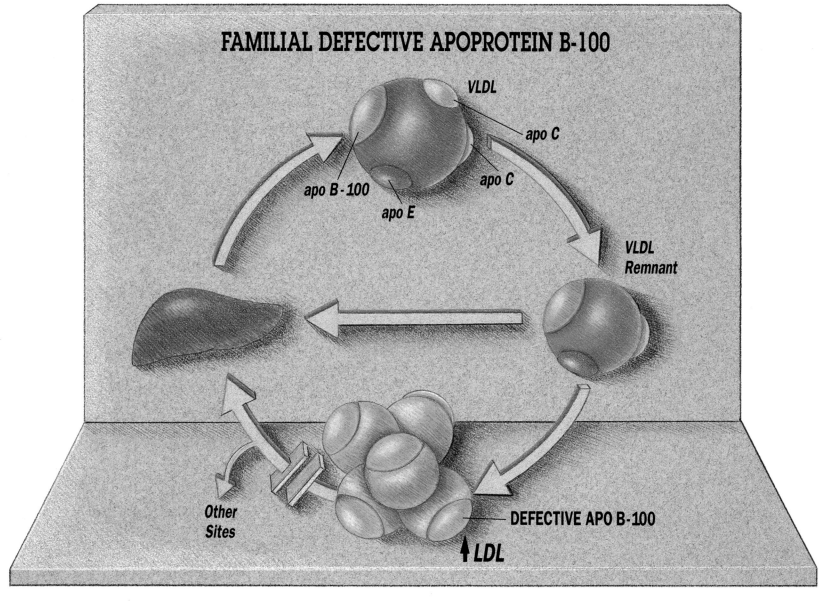

METABOLIC ABNORMALITIES RESPONSIBLE FOR POLYGENIC HYPERCHOLESTEROLEMIA

MILD DEFECTS IN LDL-RECEPTOR FUNCTION

DEFECTIVE APOLIPOPROTEIN B-100

OVERPRODUCTION OF APOLIPOPROTEIN B-100

PRESENCE OF APOLIPOPROTEIN E-4/E-4 AND E-4/E-3

INCREASED CHOLESTEROL ABSORPTION

DECREASED CHOLESTEROL CATABOLISM

HYPERRESPONSIVENESS TO SATURATED FATTY ACIDS

FAMILIAL DEFECTIVE APOPROTEIN B-100

VLDL

apo C

apo C

apo B-100

apo E

VLDL Remnant

Other Sites

DEFECTIVE APO B-100

↑LDL

Fig. 2.29 Mechanisms of familial defective apolipoprotein B-100, leading to moderate hypercholesterolemia.

cific factors affecting LDL levels have been identified (Fig. 2.28), and there is increasing evidence that they are responsible for elevated LDL levels. The term *polygenic hypercholesterolemia* is frequently applied to cases of primary moderate hypercholesterolemia that are clearly distinct from classical heterozygous FH. The word *polygenic* originally applied to the concept that several mild metabolic abnormalities combined to raise the LDL-cholesterol levels. Alternatively, the word may be considered to mean that several different defects, each of which is less severe than heterozygous FH, might separately cause a monogenic form of moderate hypercholesterolemia.

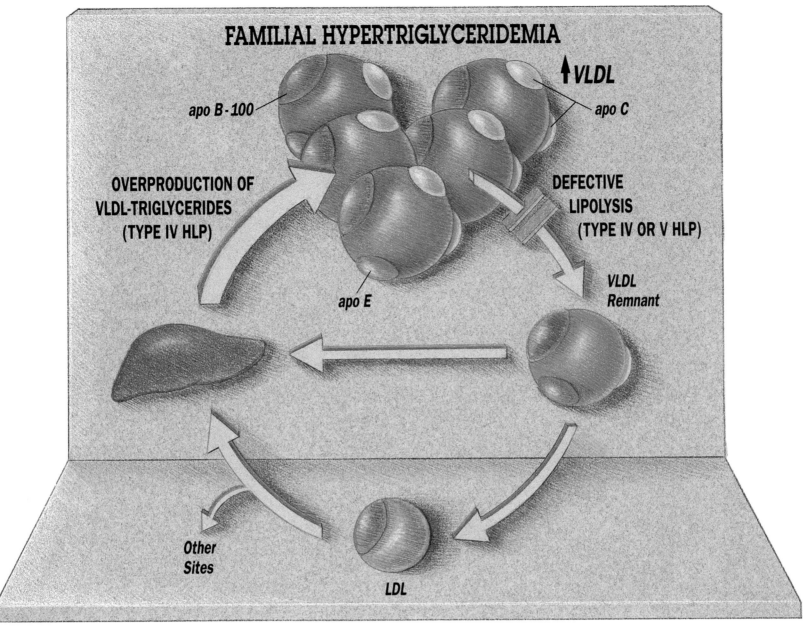

FAMILIAL HYPERTRIGLYCERIDEMIA

Fig. 2.30 Two postulated mechanisms of familial hypertriglyceridemia: overproduction of VLDL - triglycerides and defective lipolysis of triglyceride - rich lipoproteins. Both mechanisms may occur separately.

Possible abnormalities of the latter type could include mild defects in LDL-receptor function, such as point mutations in the LDL-receptor molecule; a defective apo B-100 molecule; increased synthesis of apo B-100; increased absorption or decreased catabolism of cholesterol; the presence of apo E-4 and/or an inherited hyperresponsiveness to saturated fatty acids. Any of these defects theoretically could produce moderate hypercholesterolemia.

FAMILIAL DEFECTIVE APOLIPOPROTEIN B-100

One example of an inherited defect that can cause moderate hypercholesterolemia is familial defective apo B-100 (Fig. 2.29). In this disorder, the apo B-100 molecule is defective and fails to bind normally to LDL receptors. The abnormality in lipoprotein metabolism is limit-

ed to LDL-cholesterol, since VLDL remnants having normal apo E can bind to receptors. The disorder thus differs from heterozygous FH in that uptake of VLDL remnants is normal, and hence the amount of VLDL converted to LDL is normal. This leads to a somewhat lower level of LDL-cholesterol than in heterozygous FH. The frequency of familial defective apo B-100 has not been determined, but it appears to be a relatively common cause of moderate hypercholesterolemia. Currently, its presence in a hypercholesterolemic patient can be detected only by techniques of molecular biology.

FAMILIAL HYPERTRIGLYCERIDEMIA

This disorder, which is characterized by the monogenic inheritance of pure hypertriglyceridemia, often is not expressed in childhood, becoming mani-

fest only in adults. Serum triglyceride levels are usually in the range of 300 to 800 mg/dl, and serum total cholesterol levels are typically less than 240 mg/dl. There may be more than one cause of inherited hypertriglyceridemia (Fig. 2.30). In some families, the predominant abnormality appears to be an overproduction of VLDL-triglycerides by the liver; this defect induces type IV HLP. In other families, the abnormality seems to be defective lipolysis of triglyceride-rich lipoproteins, resulting in either type IV or type V HLP. The biochemical defects underlying both abnormalities in triglyceride metabolism are poorly understood. There is a dispute whether familial hypertriglyceridemia imparts an increased risk for CHD. On the one hand, the isolated inheritance of elevated VLDL-triglycerides does not appear to be highly atherogenic; but on the other, the metabolic consequences of hypertriglyceridemia

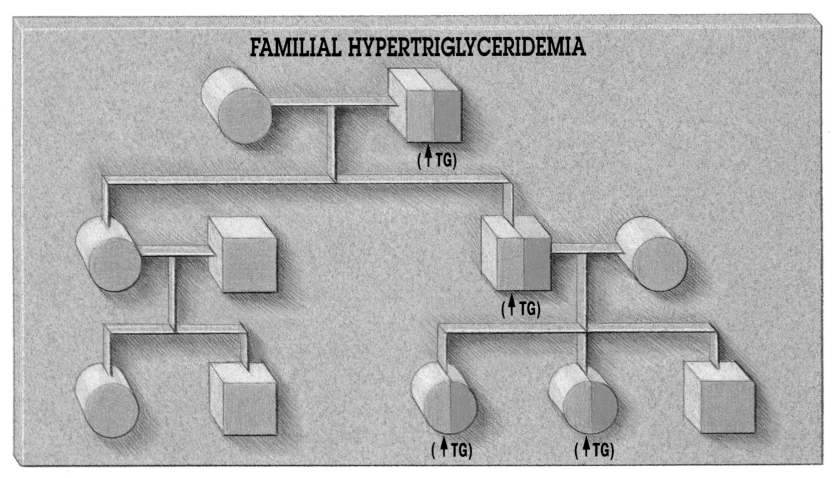

Fig. 2.31 Inheritance of familial hypertriglyceridemia as a monogenic-dominant disorder.

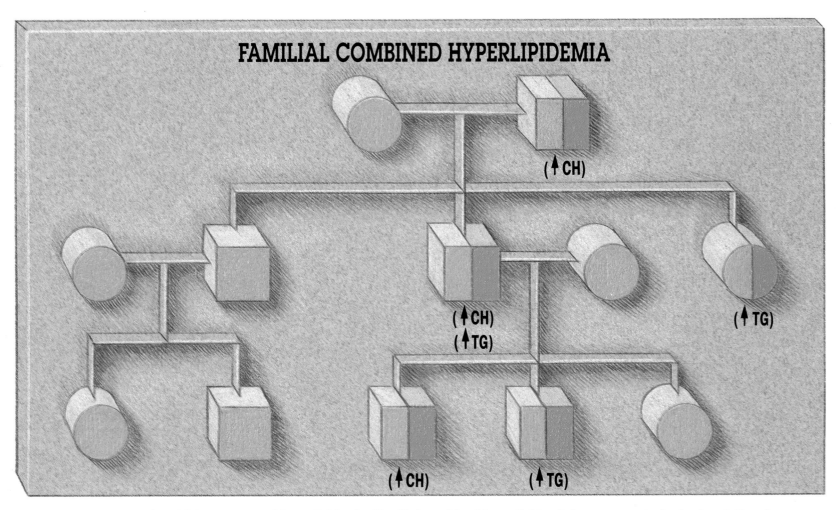

Fig. 2.32 Inheritance of multiple patterns of hyperlipidemia (familial combined hyperlipidemia) as a monogenic-dominant disorder.

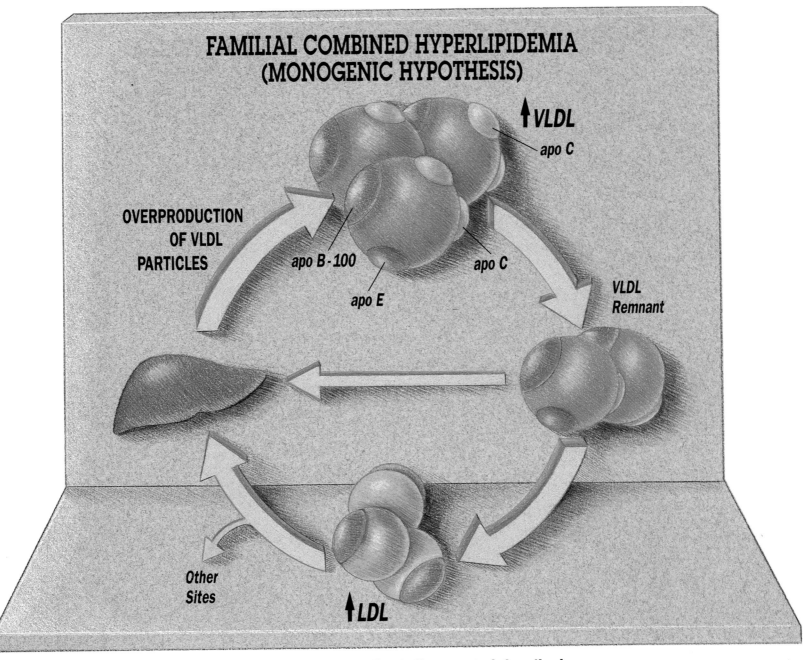

FAMILIAL COMBINED HYPERLIPIDEMIA (MONOGENIC HYPOTHESIS)

↑VLDL

apo C

OVERPRODUCTION
OF VLDL
PARTICLES

apo B-100

apo C

apo E

VLDL
Remnant

Other
Sites

↑LDL

Fig. 2.33 Mechanism of familial combined hyperlipidemia according to the monogenic hypothesis.

may increase coronary risk (see Fig. 2.12). The diagnosis of familial hypertriglyceridemia can be made only by family screening, i.e., by detection of isolated elevations of serum triglycerides in approximately half of first-degree relatives (Fig. 2.31).

FAMILIAL COMBINED HYPERLIPIDEMIA

Familial combined hyperlipidemia is typified by the findings of multiple patterns of hyperlipidemia, i.e., hypercholesterolemia, hypertriglyceridemia, and mixed hyperlipidemia, in a single family (Fig. 2.32). Moreover, multiple lipoprotein phenotypes (e.g., HLP types IIA, IIB, III, IV, and V) can occur in a single family. Patients with familial

combined hyperlipidemia appear to be at increased risk for CHD, regardless of the lipoprotein pattern. With the exception of polygenic hypercholesterolemia, familial combined hyperlipidemia may be the most common form of inherited hyperlipidemia; approximately 1% to 2% of the American population appears to be affected. The disorder frequently becomes manifest only in adulthood, although affected children often demonstrate mild elevations of serum lipids. Approximately 10% of patients with myocardial infarction before age 60 come from families with familial combined hyperlipidemia.

The inherited abnormality underlying familial combined hyperlipidemia has not been determined with certainty.

Two hypotheses have been proposed to explain the occurrence of multiple lipoprotein defects in a single family. According to the *monogenic* hypothesis, the single underlying abnormality is an overproduction by the liver of VLDL particles containing apo B-100 (Fig. 2.33).This mechanism could account for the variable increases in VLDL, VLDL remnants, and LDL. However, to explain the variable nature of expression of HLP by this hypothesis, it is necessary to postulate that various secondary or dietary factors (e.g., obesity, diabetes mellitus, excess dietary saturated fatty acids and cholesterol, or drugs) modify the expression of the hyperlipidemia
. Another view, a *polygenic* hypothesis, postulates that multiple primary

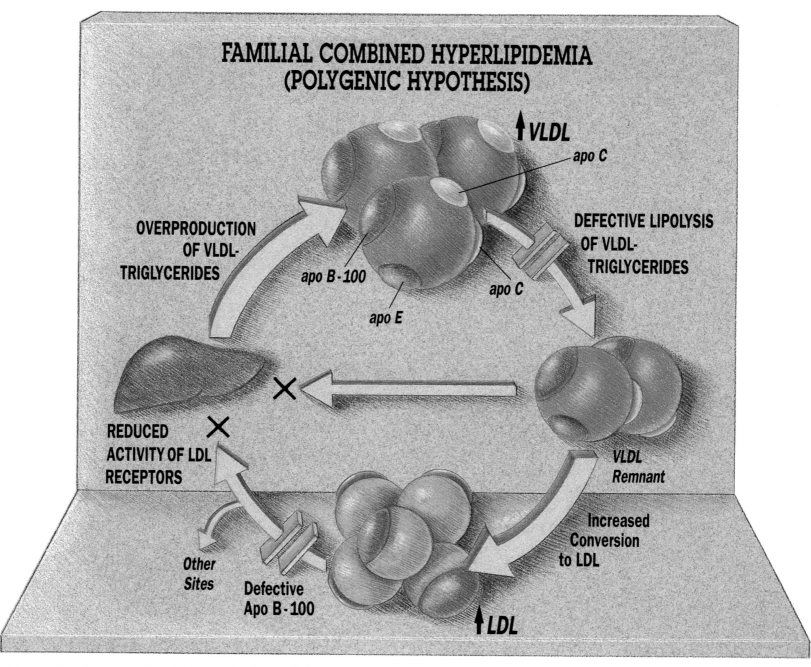

FAMILIAL COMBINED HYPERLIPIDEMIA (POLYGENIC HYPOTHESIS)

↑VLDL

apo C

OVERPRODUCTION OF VLDL-TRIGLYCERIDES

apo B-100

apo E

apo C

DEFECTIVE LIPOLYSIS OF VLDL-TRIGLYCERIDES

REDUCED ACTIVITY OF LDL RECEPTORS

VLDL Remnant

Increased Conversion to LDL

Other Sites

Defective Apo B-100

↑LDL

Fig. 2.34 Mechanisms of familial combined hyperlipidemia according to the polygenic hypothesis.

Fig. 2.35 Etiology of secondary hyperlipidemias.

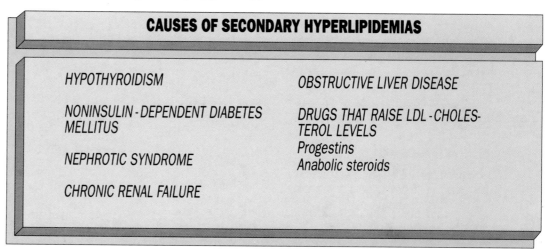

CAUSES OF SECONDARY HYPERLIPIDEMIAS

HYPOTHYROIDISM

NONINSULIN-DEPENDENT DIABETES MELLITUS

NEPHROTIC SYNDROME

CHRONIC RENAL FAILURE

OBSTRUCTIVE LIVER DISEASE

DRUGS THAT RAISE LDL-CHOLES-TEROL LEVELS
Progestins
Anabolic steroids

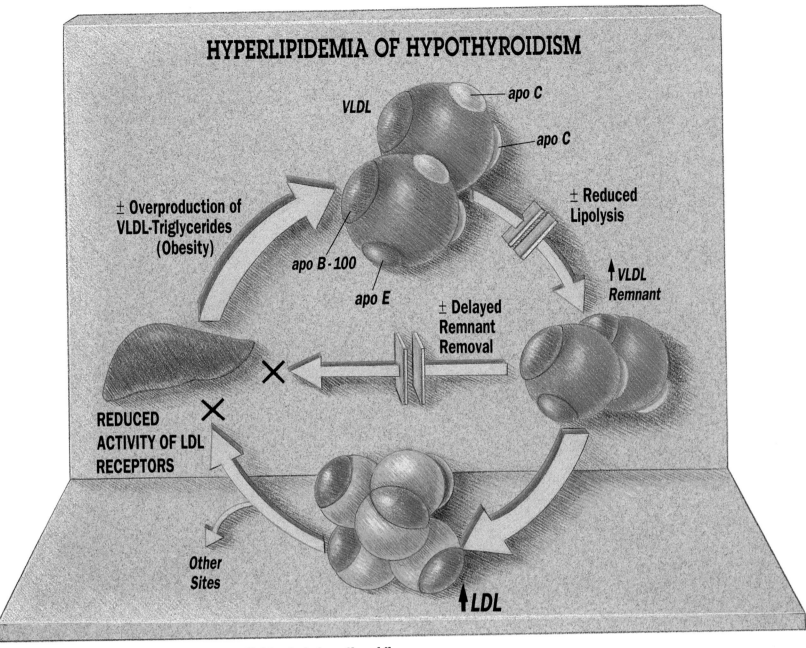

HYPERLIPIDEMIA OF HYPOTHYROIDISM

VLDL

apo C

apo C

± Reduced Lipolysis

± Overproduction of VLDL-Triglycerides (Obesity)

apo B-100

apo E

↑VLDL Remnant

± Delayed Remnant Removal

REDUCED ACTIVITY OF LDL RECEPTORS

Other Sites

↑LDL

Fig. 2.36 Mechanisms of secondary hyperlipidemia in hypothyroidism.

defects of lipoprotein metabolism are inherited simultaneously (Fig. 2.34); these defects can independently affect the metabolism of VLDL, VLDL remnants, and LDL. The polygenic hypothesis does not require the occurrence of increased synthesis of apo B-100 by the liver, a putative abnormality that has not been documented.

SECONDARY HYPERLIPIDEMIAS

Hyperlipidemia can occur as one manifestation of several diseases or as a side effect of drugs (Fig. 2.35). Hypothyroidism produces predominantly hypercholesterolemia, as does obstructive liver disease. Noninsulin-dependent diabetes mellitus and chronic renal failure induce mainly

hypertriglyceridemia. Patients with the nephrotic syndrome, on the other hand, are prone to mixed hyperlipidemia. The mechanisms underlying each form of secondary hyperlipidemia are considered below.

HYPOTHYROIDISM

The primary influence of hypothyroidism on lipoprotein metabolism is to increase the level of LDL-cholesterol, an effect that apparently is secondary to a metabolic suppression of the activity of LDL receptors (Fig. 2.36). LDL-cholesterol levels in the range 180 to 250 mg/dl are common. In addition, other lipoprotein abnormalities have been reported in patients with hypothyroidism. When these patients

become obese because of diminished utilization of energy by peripheral tissues, the excess calories can be diverted to the liver to induce overproduction of VLDL-triglycerides and hypertriglyceridemia. Reduced thyroid function may impair lipolysis of serum triglycerides, which can accentuate their elevation. Some patients with hypothyroidism, especially those with the E-2/E-2 genotype, may have delayed removal of VLDL remnants and can develop type III HLP.

NEPHROTIC SYNDROME

Hypercholesterolemia is the most common form of hyperlipidemia accompanying the nephrotic syndrome. The underlying defect, which appears to be

HYPERCHOLESTEROLEMIA OF NEPHROTIC SYNDROME

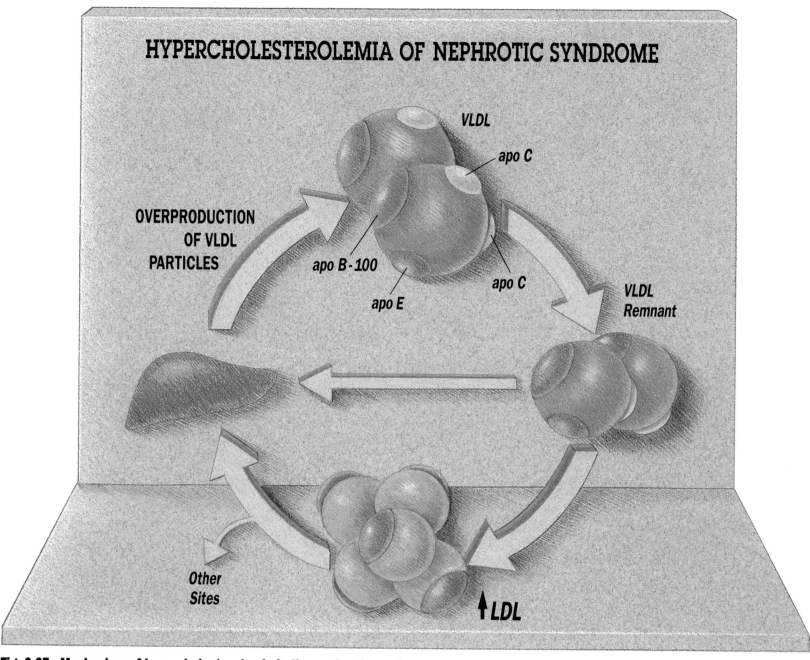

Fig. 2.37 Mechanism of hypercholesterolemia in the nephrotic syndrome.

the consequence of hypoalbuminemia, is an overproduction of lipoproteins by the liver (Fig. 2.37). This abnormality generally leads to an increased concentration of LDL-cholesterol. As the nephrosis becomes more advanced, some patients develop a defect in lipolysis of triglyceride-rich lipoproteins (Fig. 2.38); this latter change produces an elevation of plasma triglycerides. Many patients with nephrotic syndrome, therefore, have a mixed hyperlipidemia, although hypercholesterolemia usually predominates.

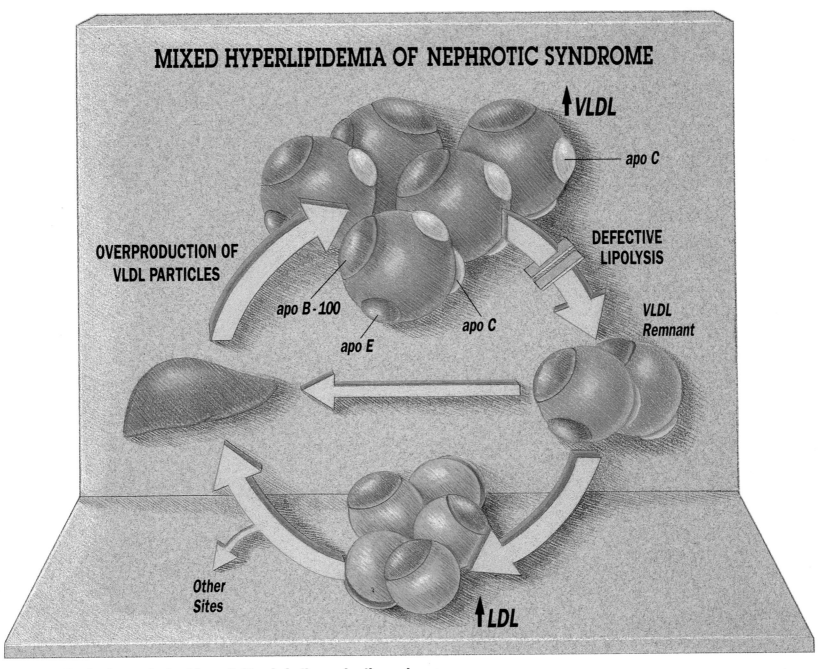

Fig. 2.38 Mechanisms of mixed hyperlipidemia in the nephrotic syndrome.

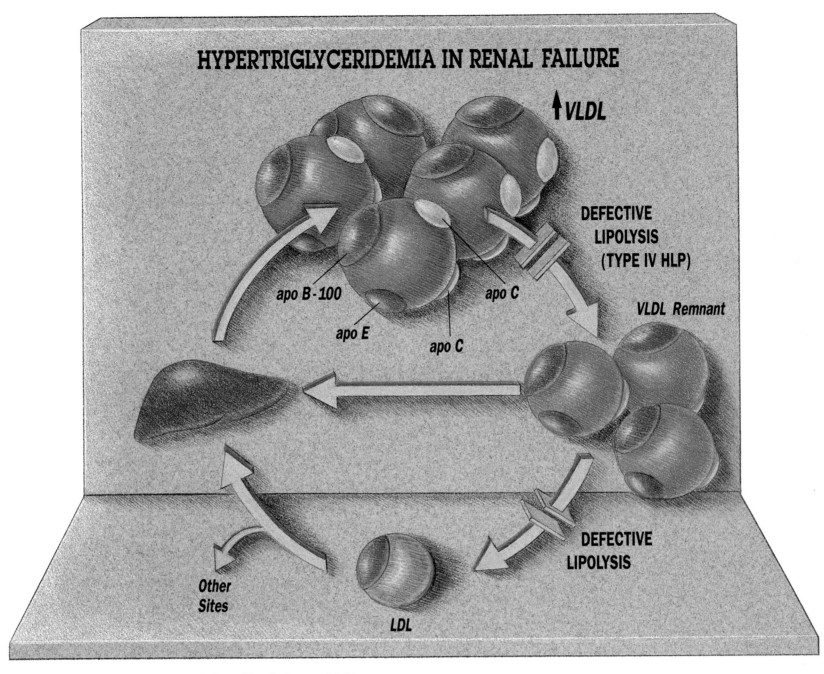

Fig. 2.39 Mechanisms of hypertriglyceridemia in renal failure.

RENAL FAILURE

At least one-third of patients with chronic renal failure have elevated triglyceride levels. The increase occurs mainly in VLDL-triglycerides, producing type IV HLP. The primary abnormality appears to be defective lipolysis of triglyceride-rich lipoproteins, which may result from an inhibition of the action of lipoprotein lipase and hepatic triglyceride lipase (Fig. 2.39). Evidence of the inhibition of both enzymes comes from the finding that LDL particles are enriched with triglycerides. Normally, residual triglycerides in VLDL remnants and LDL, remaining after the action of lipoprotein lipase, are thought to be removed by hepatic triglyceride lipase.

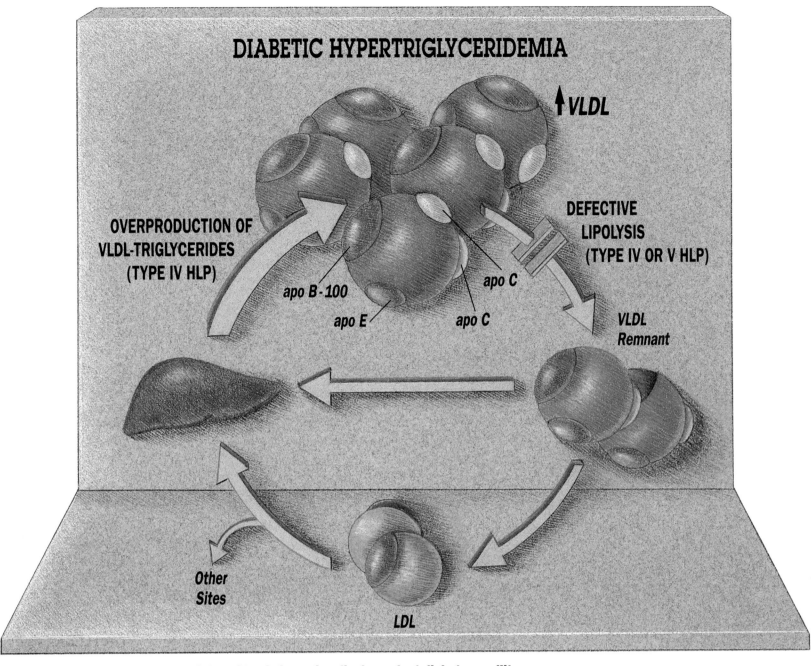

Fig. 2.40 Mechanisms of hypertriglyceridemia in noninsulin-dependent diabetes mellitus.

DIABETIC DYSLIPIDEMIA

Patients with noninsulin-dependent diabetes mellitus often have hypertriglyceridemia. Two defects contribute to elevated VLDL-triglycerides: overproduction and defective lipolysis of VLDL-triglycerides (Fig. 2.40). The former may be secondary to increased serum concentrations of free fatty acids and glucose, both of which stimulate the synthesis of VLDL-triglycerides. Defective lipolysis may result from a relative deficiency of insulin, because insulin stimulates the synthesis of lipoprotein lipase.

Unit Three

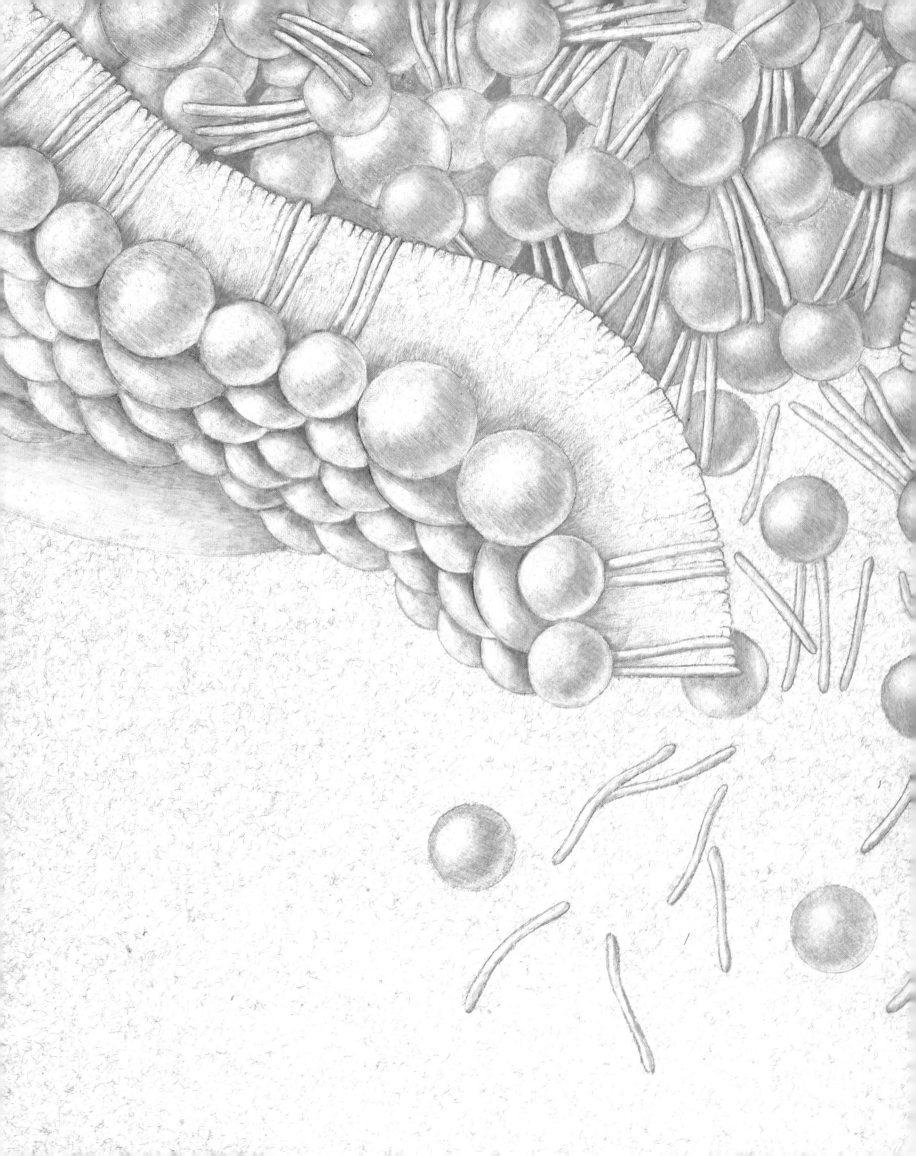

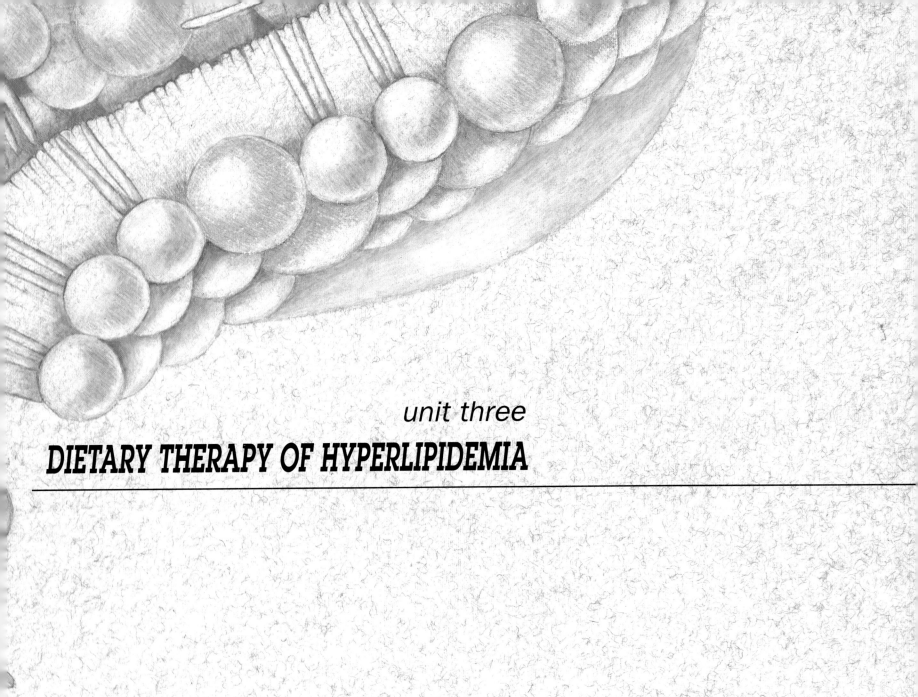

DIETARY THERAPY OF HYPERLIPIDEMIA

The high prevalence of coronary heart disease (CHD) in affluent populations has raised the possibility that environmental factors, especially diet, contribute to this disease. The diet might affect coronary risk in several ways: by adversely affecting plasma lipids and lipoproteins, by raising the blood pressure, by promoting thrombogenesis, or by precipitating the development of noninsulin-dependent diabetes mellitus. In this unit, emphasis will be placed on the influence of diet on lipoprotein metabolism as an atherogenic factor.

Three dietary factors have been identified that have adverse effects on lipoprotein metabolism (Fig 3.1). These are high intakes of saturated fatty acids and cholesterol, and excessive calorie intake leading to obesity. Another factor closely related to obesity is lack of exercise. Although other components of the diet—unsaturated fatty acids, carbohydrates, proteins, and alcohol—may affect lipoprotein metabolism, they do not fall into the category of cholesterol-raising nutrients. Each of the various types of nutrients is examined for its unique effects on lipoprotein metabolism, and then the place of each in a therapeutic diet for favorable modification of lipoprotein metabolism is considered.

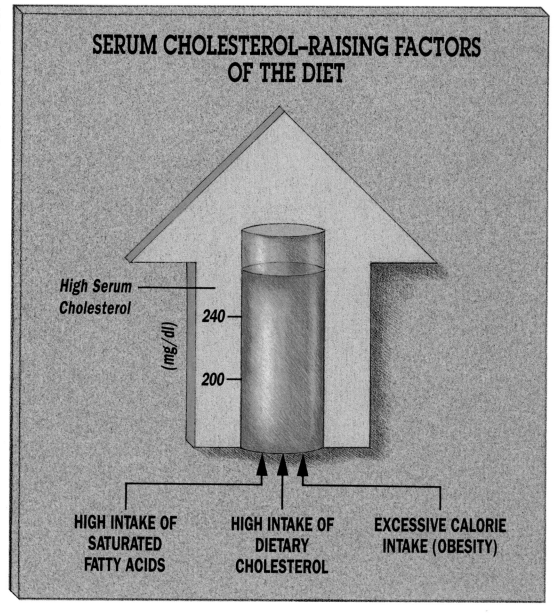

Fig. 3.1 Serum cholesterol–raising factors of the diet.

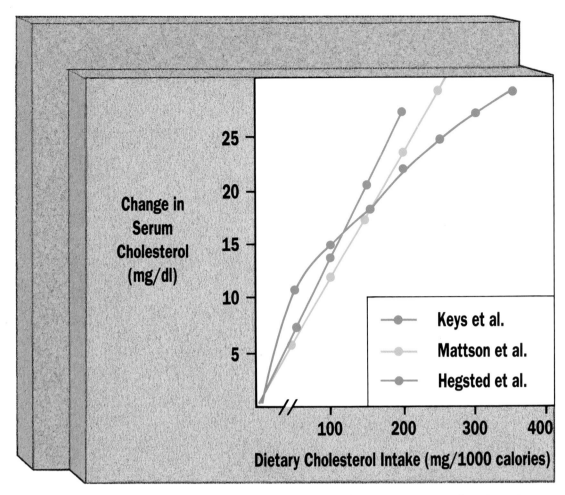

Fig. 3.2 Studies of Keys, Mattson, and Hegsted, and their colleagues, showing the relationship between increases in the cholesterol content of the diet and rises in serum cholesterol levels. (See footnote on this page for full citations of references.)

DIETARY FACTORS AFFECTING LIPOPROTEIN METABOLISM
DIETARY CHOLESTEROL

A possible link between cholesterol and CHD was first suggested by the finding that high intakes of dietary cholesterol produce hypercholesterolemia and atherosclerosis in many animal species. The degree of hypercholesterolemia thus induced is variable among species. For example, rabbits develop marked hypercholesterolemia in response to dietary cholesterol, whereas dogs and rats show a much less severe response. Many species of nonhuman primates are sensitive to dietary cholesterol and develop hypercholesterolemia and atherosclerosis with a moderately high intake of cholesterol. The sensitivity of humans to high cholesterol intake is a subject of dispute. Some workers have reported that dietary cholesterol raises serum cholesterol concentrations, whereas others have claimed that it has little or no effect. Unfortunately, many available studies have serious flaws in design that have contributed to confusion about the effects of dietary cholesterol. On the other hand, if only metabolic studies of high quality are taken into consideration, raising the cholesterol content of the diet does in fact produce a rise in serum cholesterol levels. Three studies of high quality have been carried out by Keys, Hegsted, and Mattson, and their colleagues.* The data of their studies are presented in Figure 3.2. Hegsted et al and Mattson et al found a linear relation between dietary cholesterol and serum cholesterol levels, but Keys et al found a curvilinear relationship. If these data are considered along with other available data of similar quality, it can be stated that for every 100 mg of cholesterol increment per 1000 calories per day, the serum cholesterol will increase by about 8 to 10 mg/dl.

*Keys A, Anderson JT, Grande F: Serum cholesterol response to changes in the diet. II. The effect of cholesterol in the diet. *Metabolism* 13:759–765, 1965.

Hegsted DM, McGandy RB, Myers ML, et al: Quantitative effects of dietary fat on serum cholesterol in man. *Am J Clin Nutr* 17:281–295, 1965.

Mattson FH, Erickson BA, Kligman AM: Effect of dietary cholesterol on serum cholesterol in man. *Am J Clin Nutr* 25:589–594, 1972.

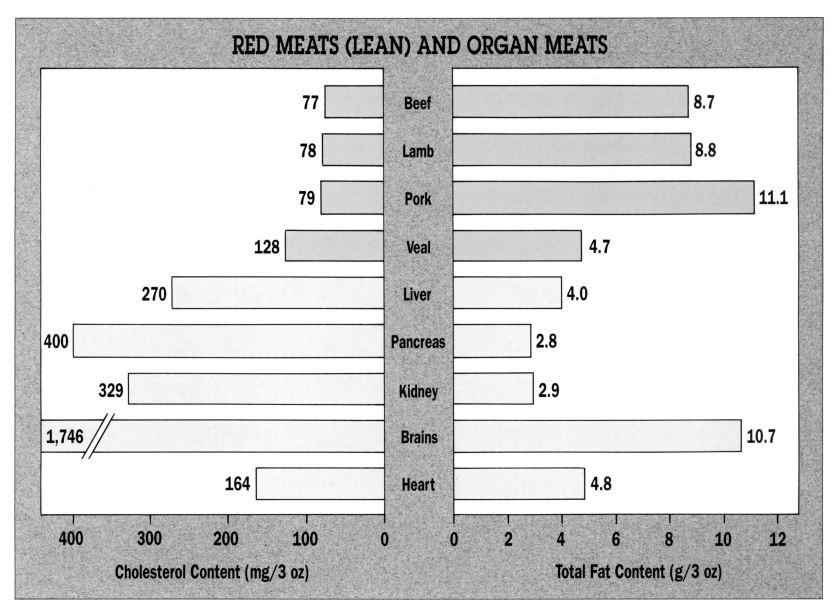

Fig. 3.3 Cholesterol content (mg/3 oz) and total fat content (g/3 oz) of lean red meats and organ meats (cooked).

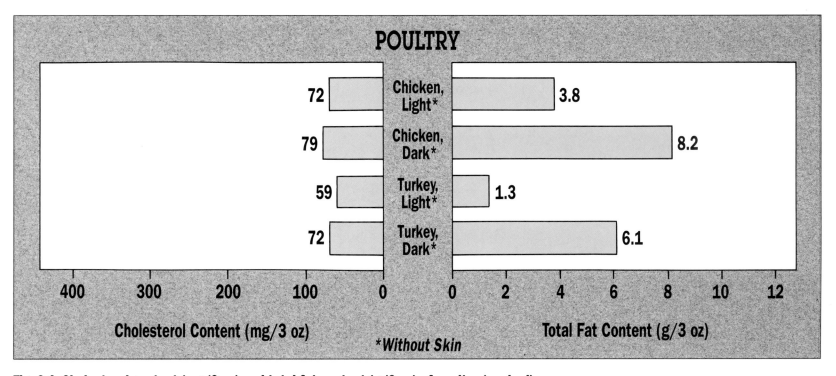

Fig. 3.4 Cholesterol content (mg/3 oz) and total fat content (g/3 oz) of poultry (cooked).

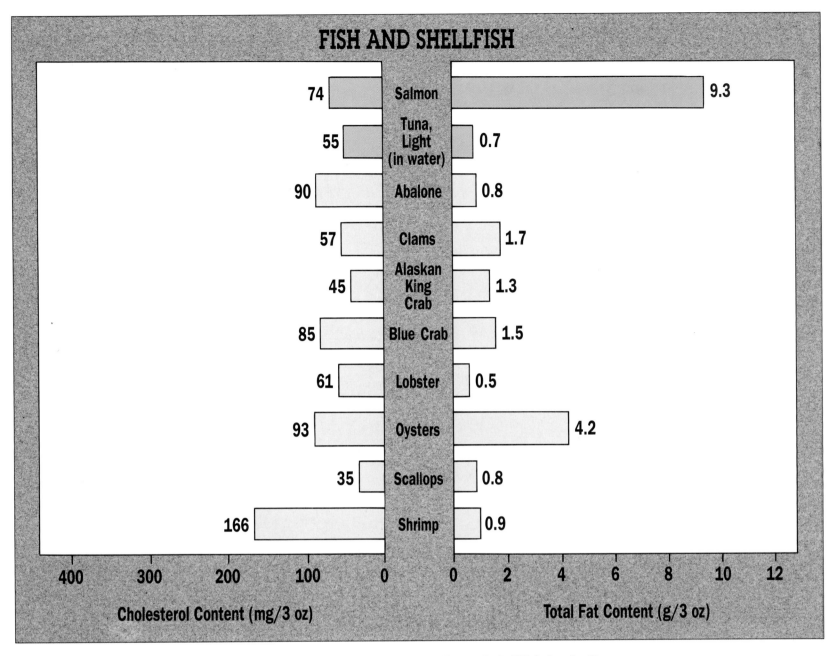

FISH AND SHELLFISH

Cholesterol Content (mg/3 oz)	Food	Total Fat Content (g/3 oz)
74	Salmon	9.3
55	Tuna, Light (in water)	0.7
90	Abalone	0.8
57	Clams	1.7
45	Alaskan King Crab	1.3
85	Blue Crab	1.5
61	Lobster	0.5
93	Oysters	4.2
35	Scallops	0.8
166	Shrimp	0.9

Fig. 3.5 Cholesterol content (mg/3 oz) and total fat content (g/3 oz) of fish and shellfish (cooked).

All dietary cholesterol is derived from animal products; plants do not contain cholesterol. The cholesterol and fat contents of various animal products are presented in Figures 3.3 to 3.5, and those of eggs and some commonly consumed dairy products in Figure 3.6 (*see next page*). The richest sources of cholesterol are eggs and organ meats. Some shellfish are relatively rich in cholesterol. Animal meats generally are not high in cholesterol, but since meat constitutes a relatively large portion of the American diet, it is still a significant contributor to dietary cholesterol. Approximately one third of the average daily intake of cholesterol comes from meat, one third from eggs,

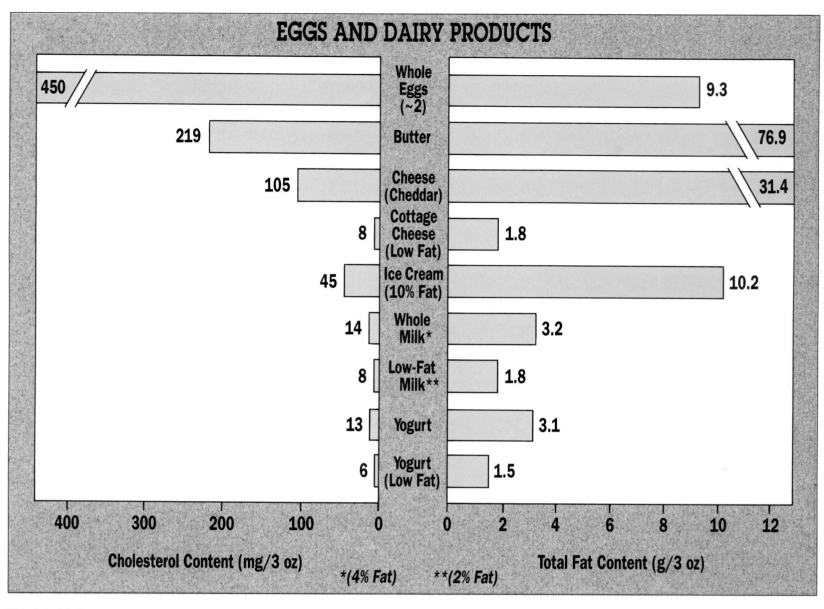

EGGS AND DAIRY PRODUCTS

Cholesterol Content (mg/3 oz)	Product	Total Fat Content (g/3 oz)
450	Whole Eggs (~2)	9.3
219	Butter	76.9
105	Cheese (Cheddar)	31.4
8	Cottage Cheese (Low Fat)	1.8
45	Ice Cream (10% Fat)	10.2
14	Whole Milk*	3.2
8	Low-Fat Milk**	1.8
13	Yogurt	3.1
6	Yogurt (Low Fat)	1.5

Cholesterol Content (mg/3 oz)　　　Total Fat Content (g/3 oz)

*(4% Fat)　　**(2% Fat)

Fig. 3.6 Cholesterol content (mg/3 oz) and total fat content (g/3 oz) of eggs and some common dairy products.

Fig. 3.7 Typical sources of dietary cholesterol.

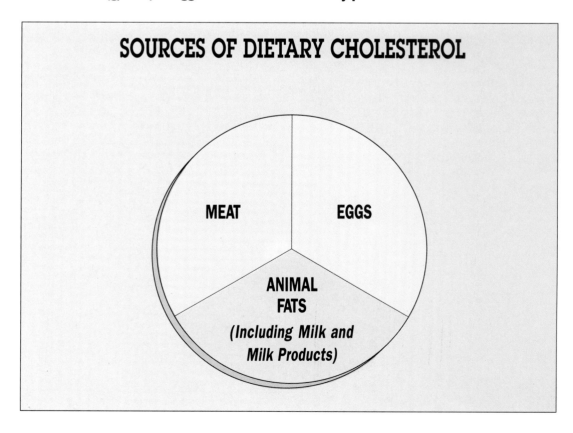

SOURCES OF DIETARY CHOLESTEROL

MEAT　　EGGS

ANIMAL FATS
(Including Milk and Milk Products)

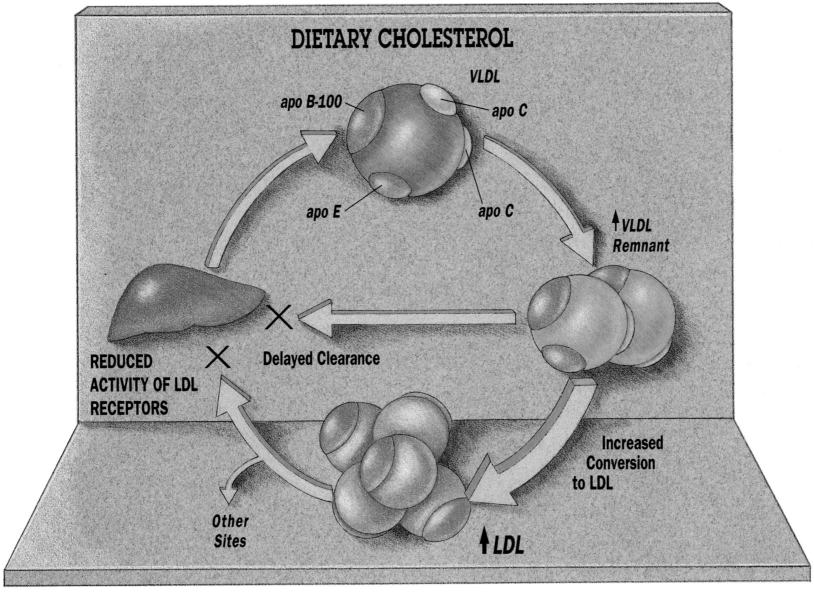

Fig. 3.8 Effects of high intakes of dietary cholesterol on the basic pathways of lipoprotein metabolism.

and one third from animal fats (including milk and milk products) (Fig. 3.7). The current intake of dietary cholesterol averages 435 mg/day for adult men, 304 mg/day for women, and 254 mg/day for children. Over the past two decades there has been a reduction in intake of cholesterol among Americans, a change due mainly to a decrease in the consumption of eggs.

The major effect of increased dietary cholesterol is to raise the LDL-cholesterol level. When increased quantities of cholesterol are absorbed, they pass to

the liver via chylomicron remnants, which increases the hepatic content of cholesterol. This leads to suppression of synthesis of LDL receptors via mechanisms described in Unit One (see Figs. 1.23, 1.25). The decrease in LDL-receptor activity raises the LDL concentration by two mechanisms: delayed clearance of circulating LDL and decreased uptake of VLDL remnants, the latter resulting in increased conversion of VLDL to LDL (Fig. 3.8). Delayed direct removal of VLDL remnants leads to an increased concentration of these lipopro-

teins as well. This rise in LDL and VLDL remnant concentrations is one mechanism whereby high intakes of dietary cholesterol raise the risk for CHD.

Several epidemiologic studies suggest that high-cholesterol diets increase CHD risk in ways beyond raising concentrations of cholesterol in fasting lipoproteins, i.e., LDL and VLDL remnants. One postulated mechanism for this "independent" effect of dietary cholesterol on CHD risk is an increase in the cholesterol content of chylomicrons and chylomicron remnants that occurs after the

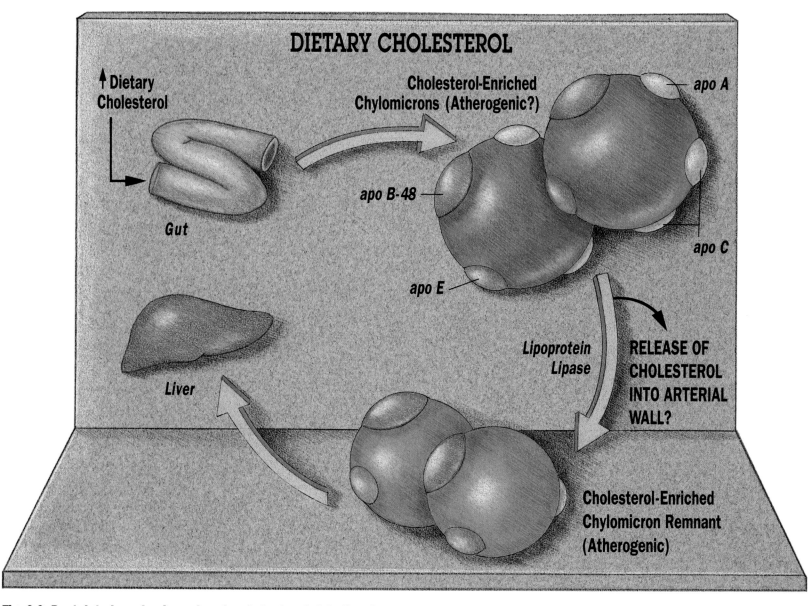

DIETARY CHOLESTEROL

↑ Dietary Cholesterol

Gut

Cholesterol-Enriched Chylomicrons (Atherogenic?)

apo A

apo B-48

apo C

apo E

Liver

Lipoprotein Lipase

RELEASE OF CHOLESTEROL INTO ARTERIAL WALL?

Cholesterol-Enriched Chylomicron Remnant (Atherogenic)

Fig. 3.9 Postulated mechanism whereby cholesterol-rich diets increase the cholesterol content of chylomicrons and chylomicron remnants, enhancing their atherogenicity.

ingestion of cholesterol-rich meals (Fig. 3.9). Chylomicron remnants are similar in size to VLDL remnants and, like the latter, appear to be atherogenic. When the diet is high in cholesterol, increased quantities of cholesterol are absorbed into the body, and this excess cholesterol might promote the development of atherosclerosis in several other ways. One possibility, for example, is that cholesterol could be lost from chylomicrons at the level of the arterial wall during lipolysis by lipoprotein lipase (see Fig. 3.9). An excess of cholesterol entering the liver from the diet could be secreted with VLDL particles and thereby enhance their atherogenicity. Even an enrichment of HDL particles with cholesterol of dietary origin could interfere with the ability of these particles to accept cholesterol from peripheral tissues, including the arterial wall; this too could enhance accumulation of cholesterol in the arterial wall. Although none of these mechanisms

has been proven, they are consistent with the concept that high intakes of cholesterol enhance atherogenesis by multiple mechanisms, and they add strength to the argument that dietary intake of cholesterol should not exceed practical limits.

SATURATED FATTY ACIDS

Several lines of evidence indicate that saturated fatty acids as a group category raise the level of serum cholesterol. Epidemiologic studies show that populations consuming large amounts of saturated fatty acids, particularly in the form of animal fats, have relatively high levels of serum cholesterol. In contrast, low intakes of saturated fatty acids in populations are accompanied by low concentrations of total cholesterol. These relationships are vividly illustrated in the Seven Countries Study (Fig. 3.10), but they have been noted in many other epidemiologic surveys.

In metabolic ward investigations, substitution of fatty acids for any other major nutrient (unsaturated fatty acids and carbohydrates) will raise the cholesterol level. The latter investigations have defined the average increase in cholesterol levels when saturated fatty acids are added to the diet. According to Ancel Keys and associates, substitution of saturated fatty acids for either monounsaturated fatty acids or carbohydrates will raise the cholesterol level by 2.7 mg/dl for every 1% of calories substituted. These workers also found that polyunsaturated fatty acids will reduce serum total cholesterol levels by 1.35 mg/dl on the same exchange with monounsaturates (or carbohydrates). These findings led to the well known predictive equations of Keys and associates, as well as to similar equations developed by Mark Hegsted and co-workers. Both equations are presented in Figure 3.11.

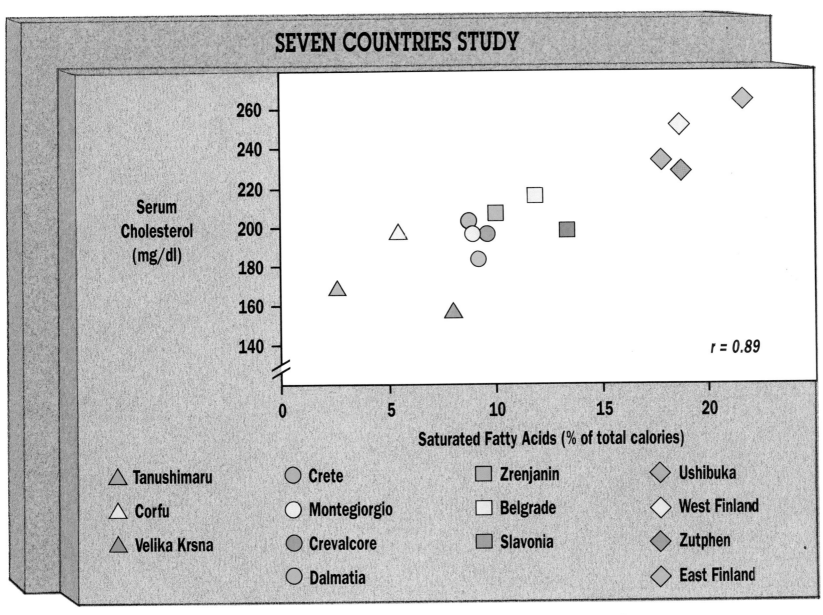

Fig. 3.10 Epidemiologic evidence showing the relationship between intakes of saturated fatty acids and serum cholesterol levels: the Seven Countries Study.

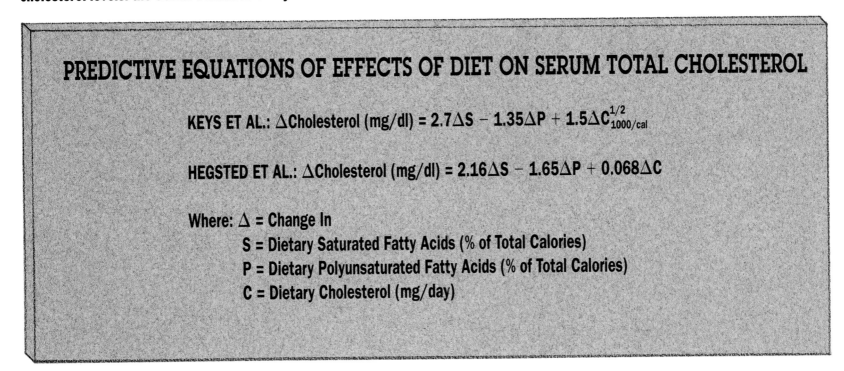

PREDICTIVE EQUATIONS OF EFFECTS OF DIET ON SERUM TOTAL CHOLESTEROL

KEYS ET AL.: ΔCholesterol (mg/dl) $= 2.7\Delta S - 1.35\Delta P + 1.5\Delta C^{1/2}_{1000/cal}$

HEGSTED ET AL.: ΔCholesterol (mg/dl) $= 2.16\Delta S - 1.65\Delta P + 0.068\Delta C$

Where: Δ = Change In
 S = Dietary Saturated Fatty Acids (% of Total Calories)
 P = Dietary Polyunsaturated Fatty Acids (% of Total Calories)
 C = Dietary Cholesterol (mg/day)

Fig. 3.11 Predictive equations of Keys and Hegsted, and their colleagues, concerning the effects of diet on serum total cholesterol.

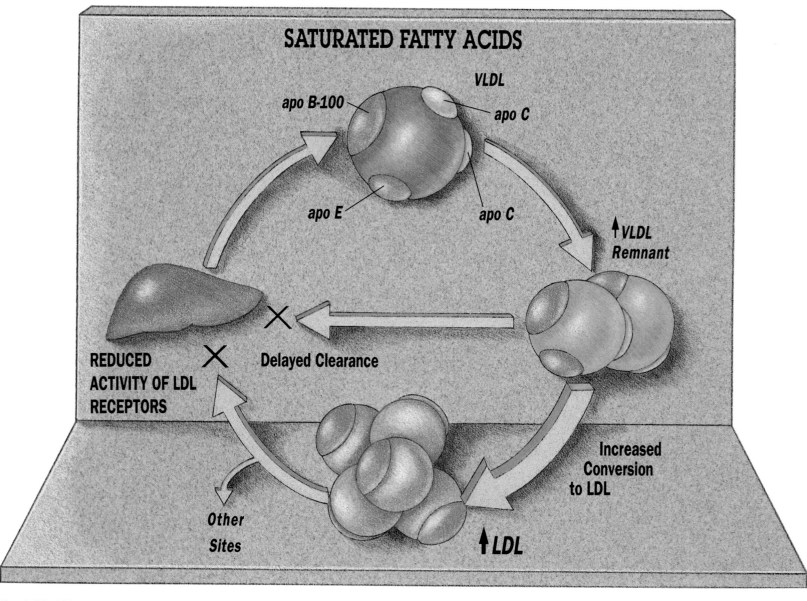

Fig. 3.12 Effects of high intakes of saturated fatty acids on the basic pathways of lipoprotein metabolism.

Fig. 3.13 Carbon-chain lengths of common saturated fatty acids of the diet.

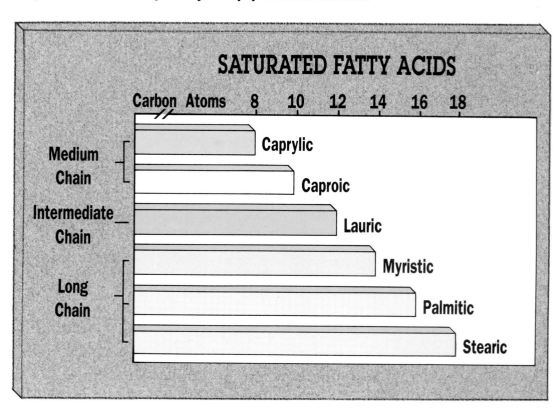

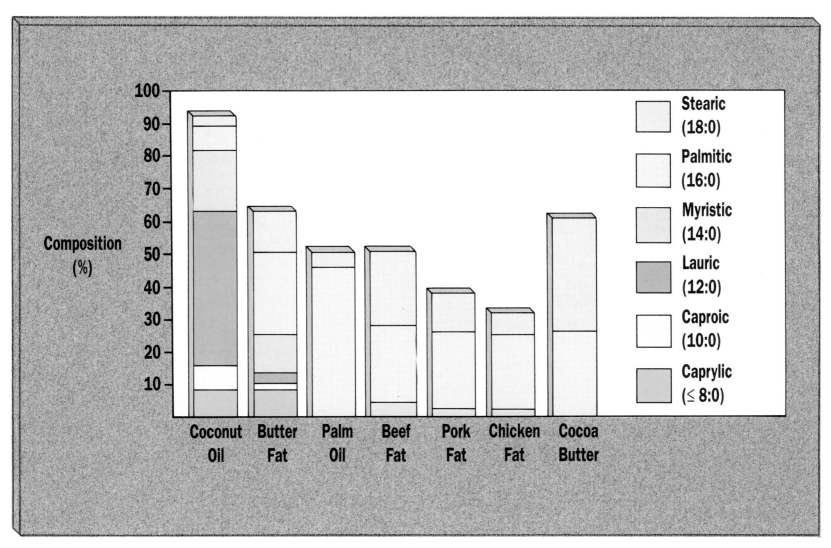

Fig. 3.14 Saturated fatty acid composition of common animal fats and some vegetable oils. The remainder of fatty acids, up to 100%, is made up of unsaturates, either mono- or polyunsaturated fatty acids.

The mechanisms whereby saturated fatty acids increase the serum cholesterol have been a subject of extensive research. Although various mechanisms have been postulated, the most likely appears to be a suppression of the activity of LDL receptors. The consequences of this reduction of LDL-receptor activity are the same as those described for the effects of diets high in cholesterol intake, namely, a delayed clearance of both LDL and VLDL remnants (Fig. 3.12). The precise means whereby saturated fatty acids suppress LDL-receptor activity are poorly understood. One possibility is that they cause a redistribution of cholesterol within liver cells, expanding the size of the metabolically active pool of cholesterol; this effect could make more "active cholesterol" available for suppression of LDL-receptor transcription (see Fig. 1.25). In fact, diets high in saturated fatty acids fed to animals have been shown to lower hepatic concentrations of messenger RNA necessary for synthesis of LDL-receptor proteins. Another

postulated effect of saturated fatty acids is to alter the composition of phospholipids in the membranes of cells so that the normal movement of LDL-receptors to the surface of the cells and their clustering in coated pits are retarded (see Figs. 1.23, 2.24). This effect could interfere with receptor binding and internalization of LDL particles. Finally, the composition of LDL particles themselves may be changed in a way that retards their binding to LDL receptors.

Dietary fats contain several different types of saturated fatty acids. They are all straight-chained organic acids, containing an even number of carbon atoms; they differ only by the length of their carbon chain (Fig. 3.13). They are represented numerically by the number of carbon atoms and the number of unsaturated links between carbon atoms (double bonds). Thus, caprylic acid (8:0) has eight carbon atoms and no double bonds. Caprylic acid and caproic acid (10:0) are called medium-chain fatty acids; lauric acid (12:0) is

intermediate, whereas myristic acid (14:0), palmitic acid (16:0), and stearic acid (18:0) are called long-chain fatty acids.

Animal fats typically are rich in saturated fatty acids, but all vegetable oils contain at least some saturates. A few vegetable oils—coconut oil, palm oil, palm kernel oil, and cocoa butter—are quite rich in saturated fatty acids (Fig. 3.14). Coconut oil and palm kernel oil have a similar composition; they are both highly saturated, but are rich in medium-chain fatty acids (8:0 and 10:0) and the intermediate-chain lauric acid (12:0). Butterfat also contains moderate quantities of medium-chain fatty acids, and it is relatively rich in myristic acid (14:0). Palm oil contains almost 50% of fatty acids in the form of saturates, most of which are palmitic acid. Cocoa butter has a similar percentage of saturated acids, but in contrast to palm oil, stearic acid (18:0) is the predominant saturated acid. Beef fat (tallow) also is high in total saturates, but it too is relatively rich in

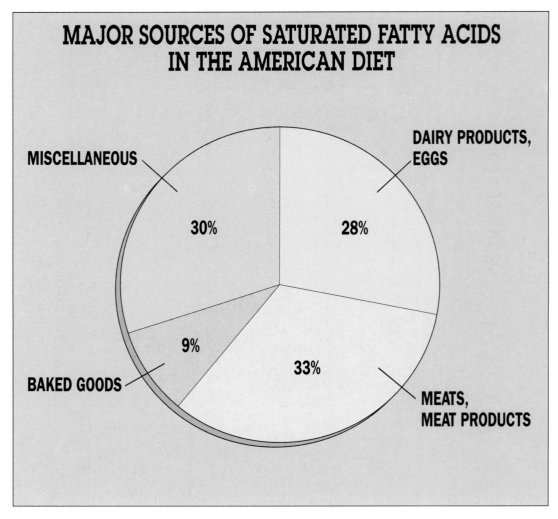

Fig. 3.15 Major sources of saturated fatty acids in the American diet.

stearic acid. Pork fat (lard) and chicken fat have lesser amounts of stearic acid, but they have similar percentages of palmitic acid as cocoa butter and beef tallow.

The sources of saturated fatty acids in the American diet are shown in Figure 3.15. Meat fat and butterfat supply most of the saturates, whereas "tropical" oils, although highly saturated, contribute much less. The individual foods supplying saturated fatty acids to the American diet (Figs. 3.16–3.19) represent targets for reducing the intake of saturates to lower the LDL-cholesterol level.

There is increasing evidence that all saturated fatty acids do not raise the serum total cholesterol (and LDL-cholesterol) to the same extent. For example, the medium-chain saturates (8:0 and 10:0) appear to be devoid of serum cholesterol–raising potential. The effect

of lauric acid (12:0) is uncertain, but most investigators believe that it can increase the serum cholesterol concentration. Without question, both myristic acid (14:0) and palmitic acid (16:0) increase LDL-cholesterol levels. Palmitic acid is by far the major cholesterol-raising saturate in the diet, and it usually is listed with lauric acid and myristic acid as cholesterol-raising saturated fatty acids.

Another saturated acid that contributes significantly to the diet is stearic acid. It is found in both animal fats and cocoa butter (see Fig. 3.14). Evidence obtained over two decades ago suggests that stearic acid does not raise the serum cholesterol level. This possibility was confirmed by a study carried out recently in our laboratory. This leaves palmitic acid, myristic acid, and possibly lauric acid as the major cholesterol-raising saturated fatty acids of the diet.

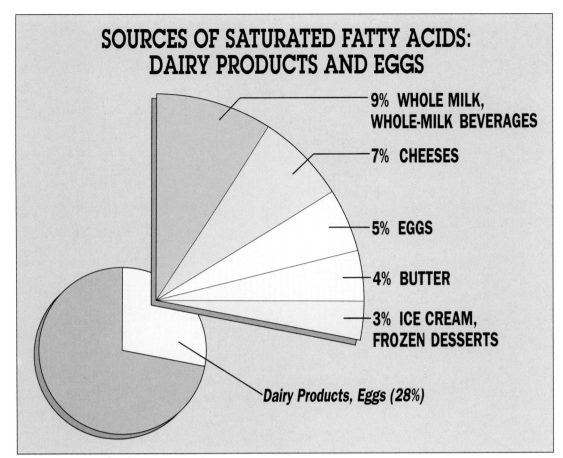

SOURCES OF SATURATED FATTY ACIDS: DAIRY PRODUCTS AND EGGS

9% WHOLE MILK, WHOLE-MILK BEVERAGES

7% CHEESES

5% EGGS

4% BUTTER

3% ICE CREAM, FROZEN DESSERTS

Dairy Products, Eggs (28%)

Fig. 3.16 Individual foods contributing saturated fatty acids to the American diet: dairy products (butterfat- and other milk-containing products) and eggs

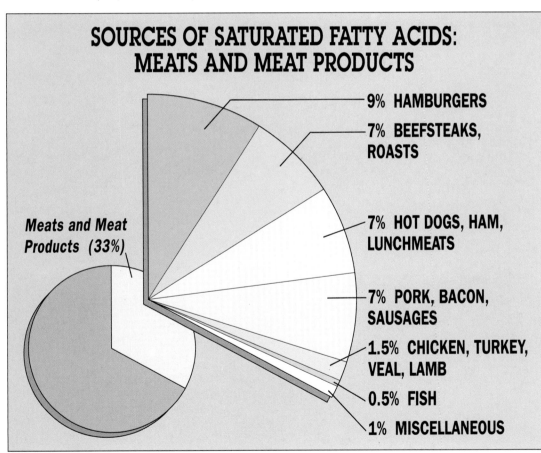

SOURCES OF SATURATED FATTY ACIDS: MEATS AND MEAT PRODUCTS

9% HAMBURGERS

7% BEEFSTEAKS, ROASTS

7% HOT DOGS, HAM, LUNCHMEATS

7% PORK, BACON, SAUSAGES

1.5% CHICKEN, TURKEY, VEAL, LAMB

0.5% FISH

1% MISCELLANEOUS

Meats and Meat Products (33%)

Fig. 3.17 Individual foods contributing saturated fatty acids to the American diet: meats and meat products.

Fig. 3.18 Individual foods contributing saturated fatty acids to the American diet: baked goods.

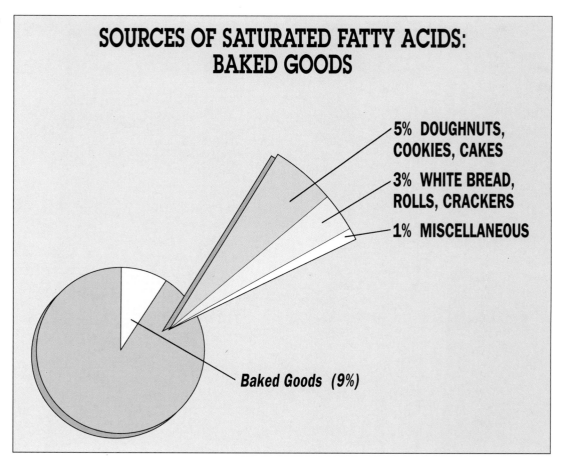

SOURCES OF SATURATED FATTY ACIDS: BAKED GOODS

5% DOUGHNUTS, COOKIES, CAKES

3% WHITE BREAD, ROLLS, CRACKERS

1% MISCELLANEOUS

Baked Goods (9%)

Fig. 3.19 Individual foods contributing saturated fatty acids to the American diet: miscellaneous.

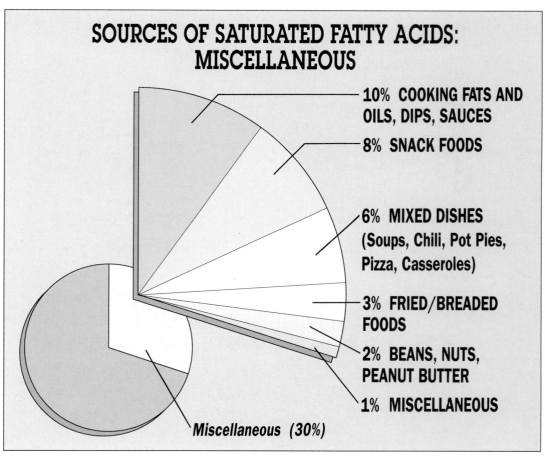

SOURCES OF SATURATED FATTY ACIDS: MISCELLANEOUS

10% COOKING FATS AND OILS, DIPS, SAUCES

8% SNACK FOODS

6% MIXED DISHES (Soups, Chili, Pot Pies, Pizza, Casseroles)

3% FRIED/BREADED FOODS

2% BEANS, NUTS, PEANUT BUTTER

1% MISCELLANEOUS

Miscellaneous (30%)

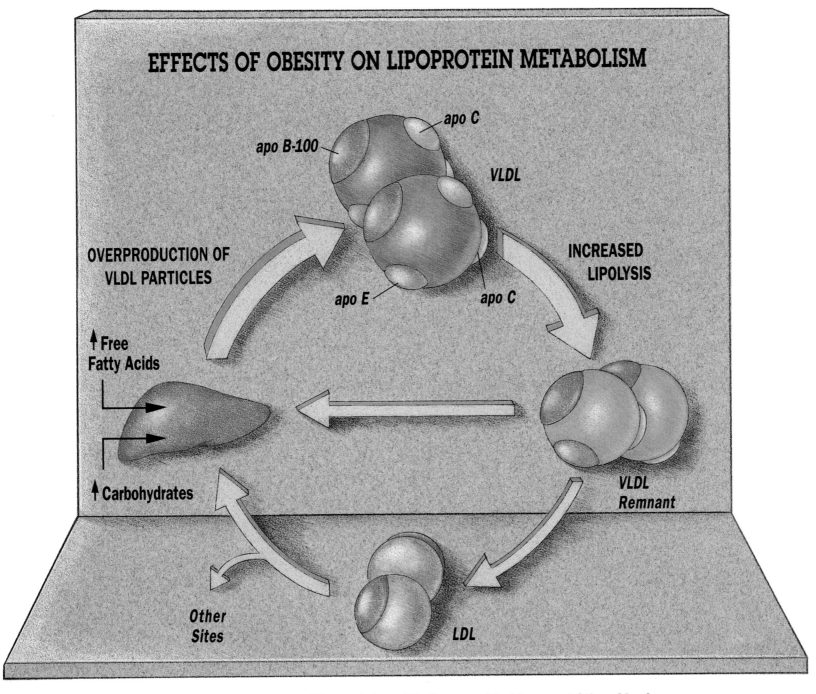

EFFECTS OF OBESITY ON LIPOPROTEIN METABOLISM

Fig. 3.20 Effects of obesity on the basic pathways of lipoprotein metabolism, resulting in normotriglyceridemia.

OBESITY

The third major dietary factor that raises the serum cholesterol is an excessive intake of total calories leading to obesity. If a high caloric intake is balanced by high energy expenditure, then obesity will not develop and consequently the serum cholesterol level will not be raised. The effects of the obese state on the metabolism of serum lipoproteins are complex, and there is not a one-to-one relationship between the degree of obesity and the serum concentrations of LDL-cholesterol. In fact, obesity can have adverse effects on all serum lipoproteins—VLDL, LDL, and HDL. Each of these effects must be reviewed to provide a complete picture of the adverse influence of obesity on serum lipids.

The major influence of obesity on lipoprotein metabolism is to induce an increased hepatic secretion of apolipoprotein B–containing lipoproteins into serum (Fig. 3.20). Evidently, the total number of VLDL particles secreted by the liver is raised in the obese state. Several elements may reinforce hepatic overproduction of VLDL particles. Foremost is an increased influx of caloric substrate into the liver. This occurs not only postprandially but also in the fasting state when surplus free

fatty acids are secreted into plasma by an enlarged body pool of adipose tissue. High serum concentrations of free fatty acids result in a heightened uptake by the liver, and this in turn stimulates the secretion of VLDL particles. This phenomenon is accentuated in the presence of visceral obesity (which is more common in men than in women) because the excess of free fatty acids released directly into the portal circulation "floods" the liver with precursors for triglyceride synthesis.

The overproduction of VLDL particles occurring in obese individuals may or may not result in hypertriglyceridemia. In general, triglyceride levels in obese

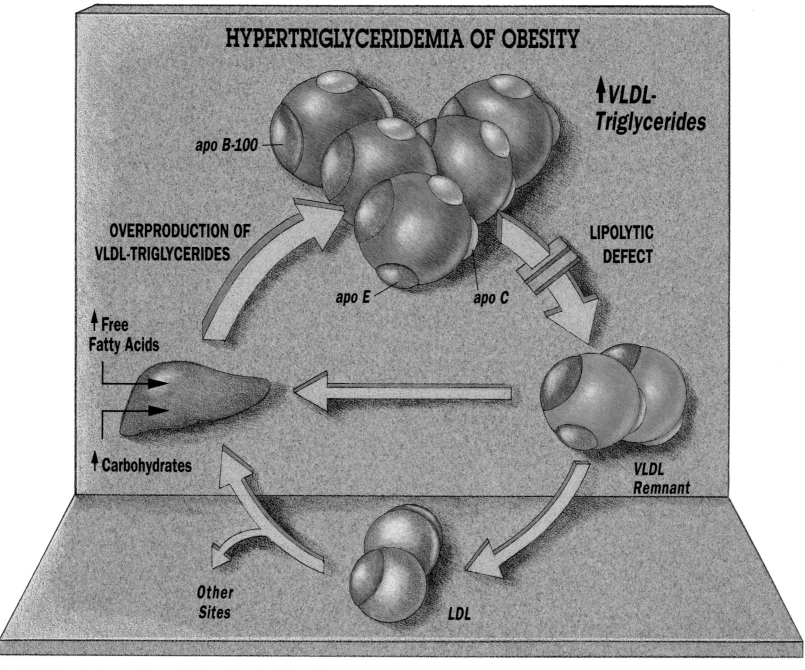

Fig. 3.21 Mechanisms of hypertriglyceridemia of obesity.

people are higher than in nonobese, and for a given individual, levels are higher than they would be if obesity were not present. Still the rise in triglyceride levels with obesity may not exceed the upper level of normal. Seemingly, many obese people have a concomitant increase in activity of lipoprotein lipase, which promotes lipolysis of VLDL-triglycerides and thereby helps maintain a normal serum triglyceride concentration (see Fig. 3.20). If for any reason a person has a relatively low activity of lipoprotein lipase or fails to increase the availability of this enzyme with weight gain, the overproduction of VLDL-triglycerides overwhelms the lipolytic system and causes an increase in serum triglyceride concentrations (Fig. 3.21). In the latter case, definite hypertriglyceridemia will result. In fact, hypertriglyceridemia is the most common serum lipid abnormality noted clinically in obese individuals. Presumably, the hypertriglyceridemia of obesity is accompanied by an increased risk for CHD because of concomitant changes in lipoprotein metabolism induced by elevated triglycerides, namely, increased levels of remnant lipoproteins, small, dense LDL particles, and reduced levels of HDL (see Fig. 2.12).

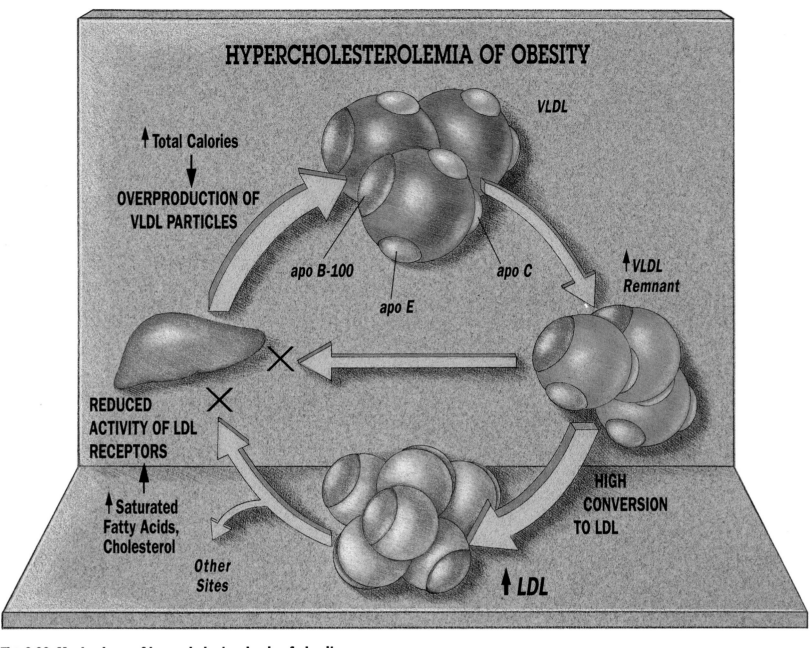

Fig. 3.22 Mechanisms of hypercholesterolemia of obesity.

Evidence is growing that the high prevalence of obesity is responsible for much of the "mass hypercholesterolemia" in the United States and other affluent societies. Two factors may contribute to this effect (Fig. 3.22). First, if the intake of saturated fatty acids and cholesterol in obese individuals is excessive, the activity of LDL receptors will be suppressed, thereby leading to a rise in the LDL-cholesterol level. Second, because of the overproduction of apolipoprotein B–containing lipoproteins in obesity, the conversion of VLDL to LDL is increased, likewise raising LDL-cholesterol concentrations. Again, however, it must be stressed that not all obese patients have hypercholesterolemia. Seemingly, some obese individuals are able to raise the activity of LDL receptors in response to obesity, and they can maintain their LDL levels near the desirable range. On the other hand, if the activity of LDL receptors in an individual is inherently low, the coexistence of obesity can induce a striking elevation of LDL levels. The importance of obesity for the causation of hypercholesterolemia in these people is revealed by the marked fall in their LDL-cholesterol values that can occur with weight reduction. Finally, if obesity produces hypertriglyceridemia, this will modify the size of LDL particles; high triglyceride levels give rise to the formation of small, dense LDL particles, which in the view of some investigators carry enhanced atherogenicity.

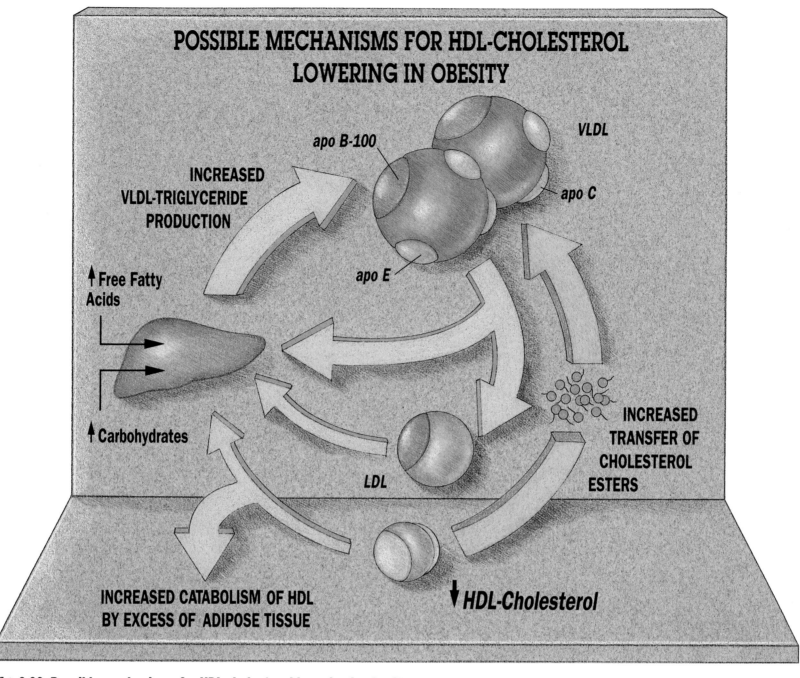

POSSIBLE MECHANISMS FOR HDL-CHOLESTEROL LOWERING IN OBESITY

Fig. 3.23 Possible mechanisms for HDL-cholesterol lowering in obesity.

Yet another effect of obesity is to reduce serum concentrations of HDL-cholesterol. The low HDL concentrations found in many obese people appear to have two origins (Fig. 3.23). First, a high concentration of triglycerides, which is common in obesity, reduces HDL-cholesterol levels (see Fig. 2.12). In addition, obesity itself appears to lower HDL concentrations independent of triglyceride levels, an effect that may be due to increased catabolism of HDL constituents by an excess of adipose tissue. When obese patients begin to restrict their calorie intake, their HDL-cholesterol levels may rise slightly as a result of the fall in triglycerides, but HDL levels do not return to normal until after a much longer period of weight reduction (i.e., until the body weight is reduced to

near the desirable range). In general, obesity causes a 5 to 10 mg/dl reduction in HDL-cholesterol levels in most individuals.

The adverse effects of obesity on lipoprotein levels are not necessarily related to the severity of obesity. Mild obesity, for example, may induce significant dyslipidemia in some people, whereas severe obesity may have little effect in others. Thus, there is a strong interactive effect between obesity and an individual's genetic regulation of lipoprotein metabolism. Mild obesity appears to be particularly detrimental in men when the excess body fat accumulates in the abdomen. This visceral obesity is particularly likely to produce elevated serum triglycerides and cholesterol and low levels of HDL-cholesterol.

The adverse influence of obesity on lipoprotein metabolism can be reversed by weight reduction. In many obese individuals, dyslipidemia will disappear following weight reduction. However, if there is an underlying genetic dyslipidemia, weight reduction alone may not completely normalize a patient's lipoprotein profile, although in most cases weight reduction will mitigate the severity of the dyslipidemia.

UNSATURATED FATTY ACIDS

The unsaturated fatty acids of the diet fall under two major categories—monounsaturates and polyunsaturates. Monounsaturated fatty acids have a single double bond in their long carbon chains; polyunsaturates in contrast have two or more double bonds. Some

UNSATURATED FATTY ACIDS OF THE DIET

FATTY ACID	DESIGNATION
Omega-9	
Oleic acid	18:1ω9
Omega-6	
Linoleic acid	18:2ω6
Omega-3	
Linolenic acid	18:3ω3
Eicosapentaenoic acid (EPA)	20:5ω3
Docosahexaenoic acid (DHA)	22:6ω3

Fig. 3.24 Unsaturated fatty acids of the diet.

common unsaturated fatty acids in the diet are shown in Figure 3.24. Among the polyunsaturates, linoleic acid is the most abundant in commonly consumed foods. Linoleic acid is an 18-carbon, long-chain fatty acid with two double bonds. One double bond is located six carbon atoms removed from the terminal carbon atom; hence, it is called an omega-6 unsaturated fatty acid. Other long-chain polyunsaturates have one double bond located in the omega-3 position. The parent fatty acid of this latter class is linolenic acid, which has 18 carbon atoms and three double bonds (18:3ω3). In the body, linolenic acid can be elongated to 20 carbon atoms and have more double bonds added; the best known in this class are eicosapentaenoic acid (EPA) (20:5ω3) and docosahexaenoic acid (DHA) (22:6ω3). Finally, the major monounsaturated fatty acid is oleic acid, which has 18 carbon atoms and one double bond located in the omega-9 position (18:1ω9). The effects of each of these categories of fatty acids on cholesterol and lipoprotein metabolism are discussed below.

Polyunsaturated Fatty Acids
Omega-6 Polyunsaturates. For many years, linoleic acid was thought to have a unique serum cholesterol–lowering action. This perceived action is indicated by the polyunsaturated fatty acid element in the equations of Keys, Hegsted, and their co-workers (see Fig. 3.11). The polyunsaturated fatty acid factor of these equations essentially represents linoleic acid. According to these equations, linoleic acid lowers the serum total cholesterol level about half as much as saturated fatty acids raise the level. Since the formulation of these equations, many nutritionists have con-

sidered the polyunsaturated/saturated fatty acid (P/S) ratio of the dietary fat to be an important determinant of the serum cholesterol concentration. The value of this ratio probably has been overemphasized. It must be noted that the equations shown in Figure 3.11 pertain to the serum total cholesterol and not to any lipoprotein fraction. Although it was widely assumed that linoleic acid uniquely lowers the LDL-cholesterol level, as it does the level of total cholesterol, this was not proven by experimentation.

In the development of the equations of Keys and Hegsted, the investigators postulated that two other major dietary constituents—monounsaturated fatty acids and carbohydrates—have no effect on serum cholesterol concentrations. In other words, they were considered to be "neutral," neither raising nor lowering the cholesterol level. Thus, the changes in total cholesterol levels attributed to saturated fatty acids and linoleic acid are relative to a zero baseline of monounsaturates and carbohydrates.

A question that has evoked considerable interest in the field of nutrition is how linoleic acid lowers the cholesterol level. Several mechanisms have been proposed. Some investigators have claimed that linoleic acid promotes excretion of cholesterol (and its products, the bile acids) from the body, thus reducing body stores of cholesterol. Others doubt this mechanism, suggesting instead that polyunsaturates cause a "redistribution" of cholesterol between the serum and tissues. Still others suggest that polyunsaturates reduce the "cholesterol-carrying" capacity of LDL, and consequently the amount of cholesterol in every LDL particle is de-

OMEGA-6 POLYUNSATURATED FATTY ACIDS

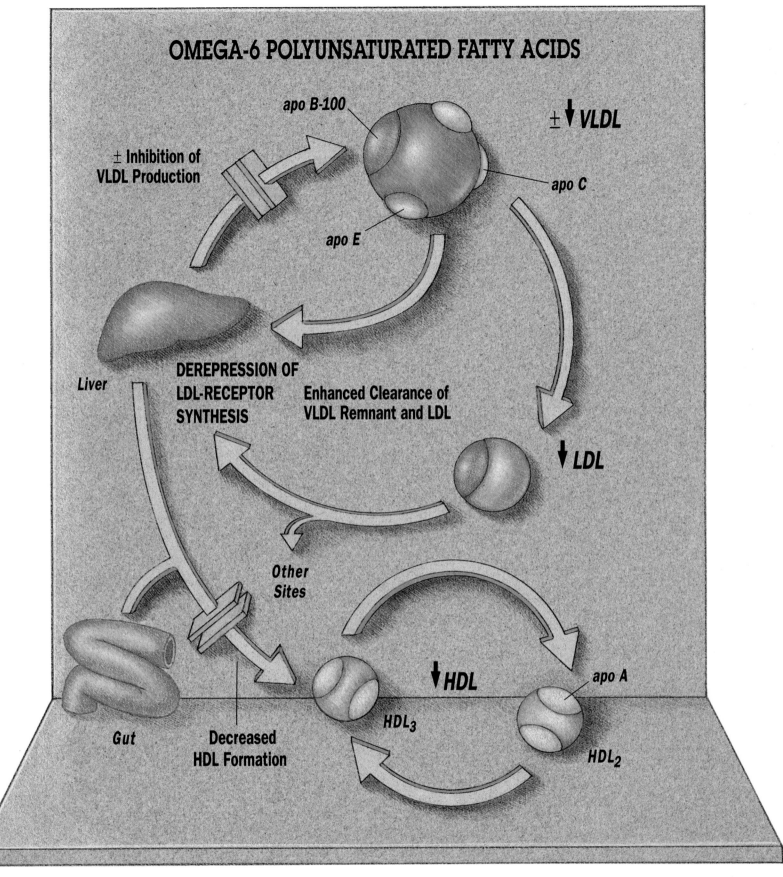

Fig. 3.25 Major actions of omega-6 polyunsaturated fatty acids (linoleic acid) on lipoprotein metabolism, resulting in a lowering of serum total cholesterol.

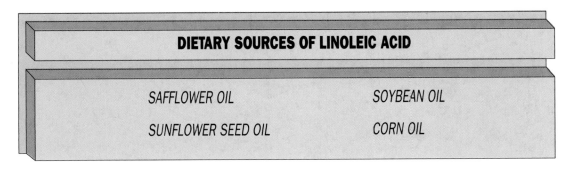

Fig. 3.26 Dietary sources of linoleic acid.

creased. The best available data, however, imply that the major action of polyunsaturated fatty acids is to increase the number of LDL receptors. Even if this is true, it is difficult to know whether the increase in number of LDL receptors that results from the exchange of linoleic acid for saturated fatty acids is due to a "cholesterol-lowering" action of linoleic acid or to removal of the "cholesterol-raising" effect of saturated fatty acids. Actually, the equations of Keys and Hegsted suggest that both of these possibilities are at work. The increase in cholesterol level from the point of neutrality (indicated by the effect of monounsaturated fatty acids and carbohydrates) has been considered to be due to the "cholesterol-raising" action of saturates, whereas the fall in cholesterol level below this "neutral point" is due to the "cholesterol-lowering" action of linoleic acid.

If linoleic acid does lower the serum cholesterol below the "neutrality" produced by monounsaturated fatty acids, in which lipoprotein fraction does this extra lowering reside? Several reports suggest that when linoleic acid is substituted for dietary saturated fatty acids, levels of VLDL-triglycerides can fall. This response does not occur universally, but when it does, there is a corresponding decline in VLDL-cholesterol. Thus, one effect of linoleic acid may be to lower VLDL-cholesterol levels, which could be secondary to a reduced hepatic secretion of VLDL. A similar lowering of VLDL-triglycerides has not been reported for monounsaturated fatty acids. A second action of high intakes of linoleic acid is a reduction in HDL-cholesterol concentrations, an effect that has been reported in several studies. Seemingly, high intakes of linoleic acid reduce the formation of HDL. Once again, an HDL-lowering action has not been reported for monoun-

saturated fatty acids. Finally, it has been believed for many years that linoleic acid has a unique LDL-lowering action. Recently, however, several reports suggest that replacement of saturated fatty acids with either linoleic acid or oleic acid produces essentially the same decrease in LDL-cholesterol levels. Therefore, the unique cholesterol-lowering action of linoleic acid may occur mainly in the VLDL- and HDL-cholesterol fractions, and not in the LDL fraction. It must be noted that the HDL-lowering action of linoleic acid occurs only at relatively high intakes; at intakes of less than 10% of total calories, such an action usually is not manifest.

The major actions of linoleic acid on lipoprotein metabolism that cause a lowering of serum total cholesterol are summarized in Figure 3.25. In some patients, linoleic acid interferes with secretion of VLDL, thereby lowering VLDL-cholesterol concentrations. High intakes of linoleic acid also reduce HDL-cholesterol levels by retarding formation of HDL. And substitution of this polyunsaturated fatty acid for saturated fatty acids leads to derepression of LDL-receptor synthesis, causing a fall in LDL-cholesterol concentrations.

The major sources of linoleic acid in the diet are vegetable oils (Fig. 3.26). These include safflower oil, sunflower seed oil, soybean oil, and corn oil, all of which are low in cholesterol-raising saturated fatty acids. Although these vegetable oils have very little LDL-raising potential as a result of their low content of saturated fatty acids, they are still high in total calories (as are all fats and oils), and therefore they can raise the LDL level if they are consumed in excessive amounts and produce weight gain.

Omega-3 Polyunsaturates. Recent interest has centered on the omega-3 polyunsaturated fatty acids found in fish oils. The major polyunsaturates in

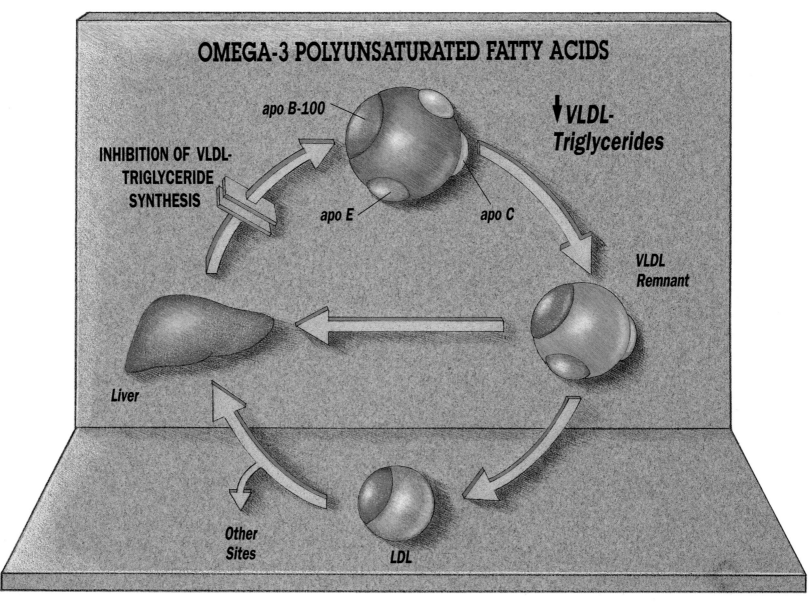

OMEGA-3 POLYUNSATURATED FATTY ACIDS

apo B-100

INHIBITION OF VLDL-
TRIGLYCERIDE
SYNTHESIS

apo E

apo C

↓VLDL-
Triglycerides

VLDL
Remnant

Liver

Other
Sites

LDL

Fig. 3.27 Major actions of omega-3 polyunsaturated fatty acids on the basic pathways of lipoprotein metabolism.

fish oils are EPA and DHA. Primarily, they act to lower serum triglycerides by inhibiting the synthesis of triglycerides in the liver (Fig. 3.27). Apparently, omega-3 polyunsaturates do not reduce the number of VLDL particles being secreted by the liver but rather decrease the triglyceride content of these particles. In other words, they curtail the input of large, triglyceride-rich VLDL, replacing them with smaller VLDL particles about the size of VLDL remnants. Consequently, ingestion of fish oils does not lower LDL concentrations except as their polyunsaturated fatty acids replace saturated fatty acids in the diet. In other words, mere supplementation of the diet with fish oils will not lower LDL levels. In patients with hypertriglyceridemia, omega-3 polyunsaturates will reduce triglyceride concentrations, but at the same time they often raise LDL-cholesterol levels. Therefore, their utility in the diet for favorably modifying serum lipoproteins

in either hypercholesterolemic or hypertriglyceridemic individuals is open to question.

On the other hand, fish oils may be beneficial for the prevention of CHD or its complications independent of their actions on plasma lipoproteins. Like aspirin, for instance, they interfere with platelet aggregation and thereby may help prevent coronary thrombosis. A limited number of studies further suggest that they may retard proliferation of fibroblasts and smooth muscle cells in response to an injury within the arterial wall; although potentially beneficial, this effect has not been proven with certainty. A recent report indicates that high intakes of fish oils reduce the likelihood of restenosis of coronary arteries following coronary angioplasty, but this putative action too requires confirmation. Overall, the omega-3 polyunsaturates are promising for both primary and secondary prevention of CHD, but until benefit

has been proven through more extensive investigation, their use for these aims cannot be recommended at present.

Monounsaturated Fatty Acids
Oleic Acid. According to the equations of Keys and Hegsted (see Fig. 3.11), oleic acid is "neutral" in its effects on serum total cholesterol, neither raising nor lowering levels. This concept has generally been confirmed by studies carried out in our laboratory. Whenever oleic acid replaces saturated fatty acids in the diet, the serum total cholesterol falls to the degree predicted by the equations. Our investigations indicate that the reduction in total cholesterol occurs exclusively in the LDL fraction. Oleic acid reduces neither VLDL nor HDL, and in this regard it differs from the actions of linoleic acid. Furthermore, our investigations indicate that when either oleic acid or linoleic acid replaces saturates in the diet, the decreases in LDL-cholesterol

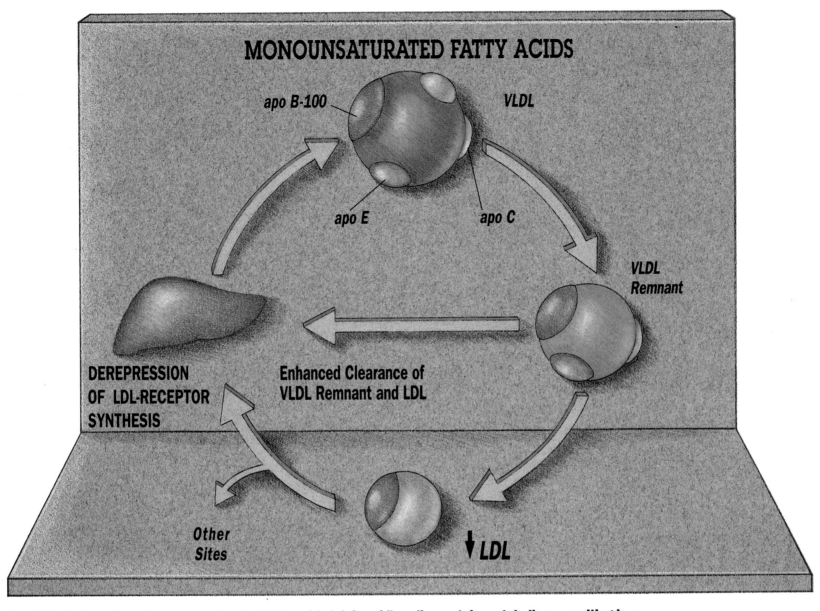

MONOUNSATURATED FATTY ACIDS

apo B-100

VLDL

apo E

apo C

VLDL Remnant

DEREPRESSION OF LDL-RECEPTOR SYNTHESIS

Enhanced Clearance of VLDL Remnant and LDL

Other Sites

↓ LDL

Fig. 3.28 Major action of monounsaturated fatty acids (oleic acid) on lipoprotein metabolism, resulting in a reduction in the LDL-cholesterol fraction.

concentration are essentially the same. Thus, our findings do not support the concept that linoleic acid uniquely lowers LDL levels beyond the reductions observed with oleic acid. Presumably, the mechanism for "LDL lowering" by oleic acid (Fig. 3.28) is the same as that for linoleic acid (see Fig. 3.25), namely the derepression of LDL-receptor synthesis.

Vegetable oils that are rich in oleic acid are olive oil, rapeseed oil (canola oil), and high-oleic forms of sunflower seed oil, safflower oil, and soybean oil (Fig. 3.29). Less commonly used oils —peanut oil, rice oil, avocado oil, hazelnut oil, and pecan oil—also are relatively rich in oleic acid. These same oils, of course, can be obtained for the diet by eating peanuts, pecans, hazelnuts, avocados, olives, and so on. Many animal fats contain large quantities of oleic acid, but most of these are relatively rich in saturated fatty acids.

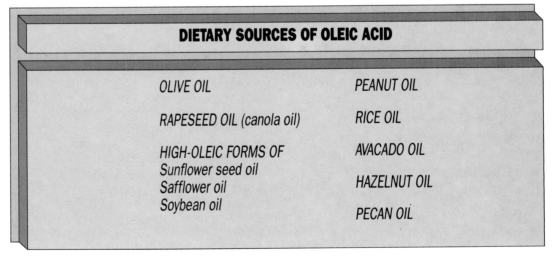

DIETARY SOURCES OF OLEIC ACID	
OLIVE OIL	PEANUT OIL
RAPESEED OIL (canola oil)	RICE OIL
HIGH-OLEIC FORMS OF Sunflower seed oil Safflower oil Soybean oil	AVACADO OIL
	HAZELNUT OIL
	PECAN OIL

Fig. 3.29 Dietary sources of oleic acid.

DIETARY CARBOHYDRATES

DIGESTIBLE	INDIGESTIBLE
Simple sugars (monosaccharides, disaccharides)	Insoluble (cellulose)
Complex carbohydrates (starches)	Soluble (pectins, gums, psyllium)

Fig. 3.30 Digestible and indigestible carbohydrates of the diet.

However, it has been shown recently that the fatty acid content of meat fat can be changed by the diet. For instance, feeding rapeseed oil (canola oil) to pigs greatly enriches their fat with oleic acid at the expense of palmitic acid.

Trans-monounsaturated Fatty Acids. When vegetable oils rich in polyunsaturates are hydrogenated, some of the fatty acids are transformed into trans-monounsaturated fatty acids. The richest sources of trans-unsaturated fatty acids, therefore, are shortenings and margarines. The actions of trans-monounsaturates on serum cholesterol and lipoprotein levels have not been studied extensively. Although several investigations suggest that they act like oleic acid and do not raise the cholesterol levels, other reports indicate a cholesterol-raising action. Consequently, more investigations are needed to determine precisely the actions of this important source of fatty acids in the diet.

CARBOHYDRATES

The carbohydrates of the diet include simple sugars (monosaccharides and disaccharides), complex digestible carbohydrates (starches), and complex indigestible carbohydrates (Fig. 3.30). The carbohydrates in the diet come mainly from fruits, vegetables, cereals, legumes, and processed foods. Normally, the diet contains between 45% and 55% of total calories as carbohydrates. Foods high in complex carbohydrates usually contain considerable quantities of vitamins and minerals. Since these foods generally are not calorically dense, relatively large amounts can be consumed without providing an excessive intake of total calories. Consequently, some investigators believe that high-carbohydrate diets are less likely to produce obesity than high-fat diets. In addition, worldwide epidemiologic studies have suggested that populations that consume low-fat, high-carbohydrate diets have lower rates of CHD and cancer than populations eating high-fat diets.

According to the equations of Keys and Hegsted (see Fig. 3.11), carbohydrates, like monounsaturates, are "neutral" in their action on the serum cholesterol level. This, however, is not to say that carbohydrates are without effects on lipoprotein metabolism (Fig. 3.31). For example, high-carbohydrate diets stimulate the synthesis of VLDL-triglycerides and thus often raise serum triglyceride levels; a corresponding rise in VLDL-cholesterol levels also occurs. At the same time, high-carbohydrate diets lower the serum concentration of HDL-cholesterol, possibly because they raise the triglyceride concentration. Removal of fat from the diet, and its replacement by carbohydrates, may further decrease the formation of HDL. Substitution of carbohydrates for saturated fatty acids reduces LDL-cholesterol levels, presumably by the same mechanism as with linoleic acid and oleic acid.

Indigestible complex carbohydrates in the diet are called fiber, which is generally classified as "insoluble" and "soluble." The insoluble fiber in the diet is mainly cellulose, as in the cellulose of wheat bran. Cellulose adds bulk to the stools, and for many people aids in normal colon function. It has been suggested that high intakes of cellulose will reduce the chance of developing diverticulitis and possibly even colon cancer. However, insoluble fibers have little or no effect on serum cholesterol levels.

The soluble fibers include pectins, certain gums, and psyllium. One example of a gum is beta-glycan, which is the predominant soluble fiber in beans and oat bran. Recent reports suggest that high intakes of soluble fibers will lower the serum cholesterol level. The mecha-

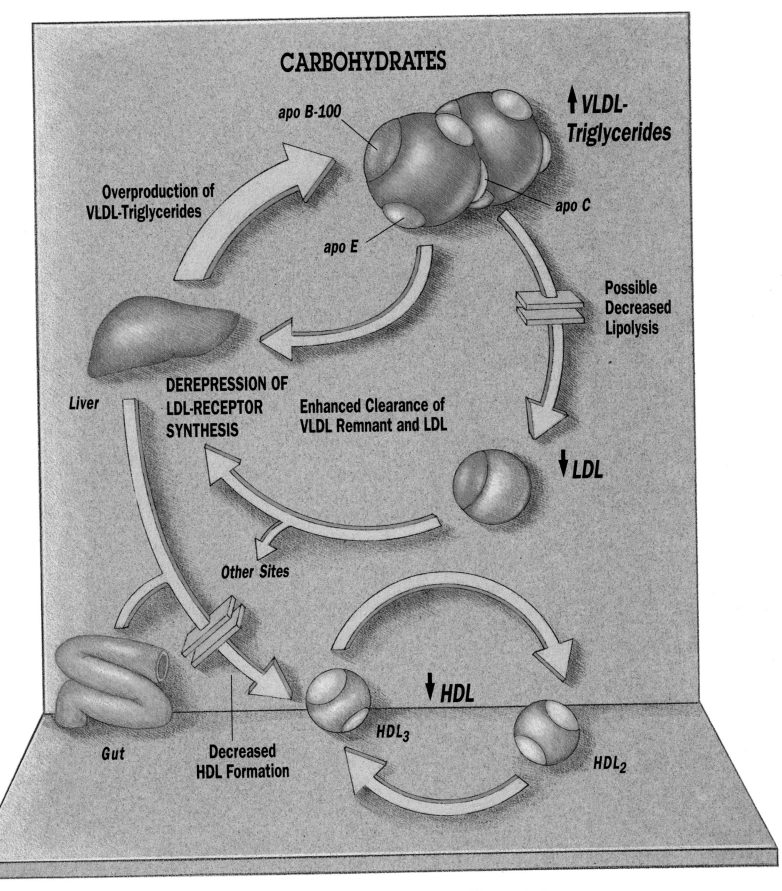

CARBOHYDRATES

apo B-100

↑VLDL-Triglycerides

Overproduction of VLDL-Triglycerides

apo C

apo E

Possible Decreased Lipolysis

Liver

DEREPRESSION OF LDL-RECEPTOR SYNTHESIS

Enhanced Clearance of VLDL Remnant and LDL

↓LDL

Other Sites

Gut

Decreased HDL Formation

↓HDL

HDL₃

HDL₂

Fig. 3.31 Major actions of a high-carbohydrate diet on the basic pathways of lipoprotein metabolism.

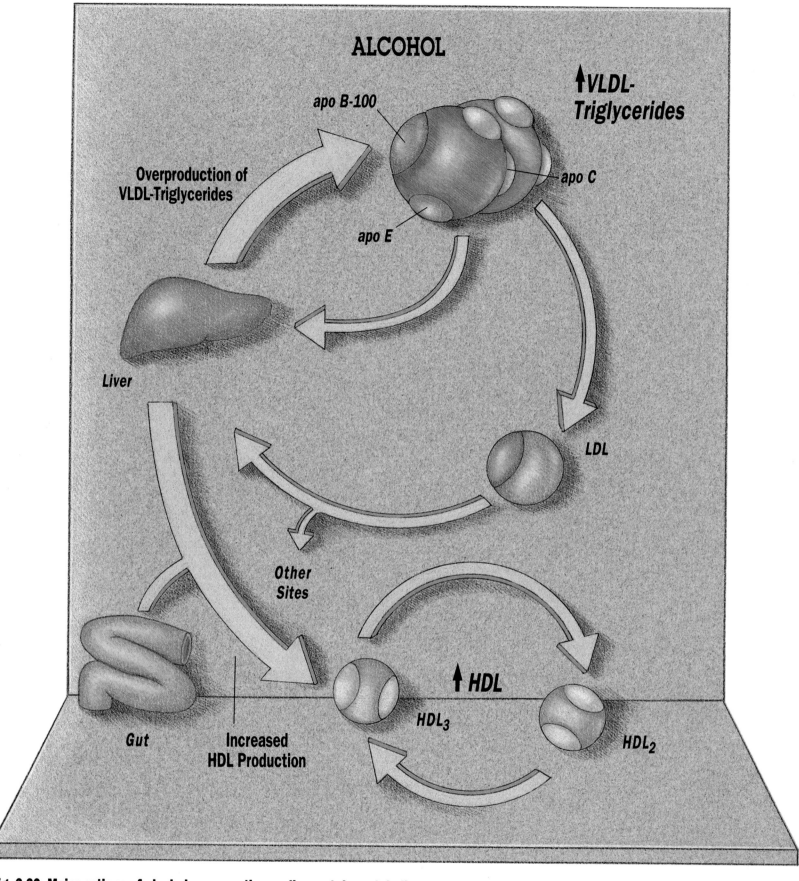

Fig. 3.32 Major actions of alcohol consumption on lipoprotein metabolism.

nism for this putative action is unknown. Although early claims of a significant cholesterol-lowering action have not been confirmed, recent investigations suggest that serum cholesterol reductions in the range of 3% to 5% may be obtained by consumption of large quantities of soluble fiber. It must be pointed out, however, that such high intakes will produce gastrointestinal side effects in many people; although prolonged usage may improve tolerance, a high percentage of people are not able to maintain the unusually high intakes required to produce a cholesterol-lowering effect.

ALCOHOL

Many Americans consume appreciable quantities of alcohol, and on the average the intake is about 5% of total calories. Some epidemiologists have suggested that relatively high intakes of alcohol may protect against CHD. This claim is based on the finding of an unexpectedly low prevalence of CHD in certain countries, notably France and Italy, where consumption of wine is relatively high. This concept is bolstered by the observation that consumption of moderate quantities of alcohol will raise levels of HDL-cholesterol, a putative "protective" lipoprotein. In spite of speculation about the possibly beneficial influence of alcohol for prevention of coronary disease, many other factors may confuse the issue, and at present there is no proof of a protective action. In individuals who are prone to hypercholesterolemia, high intakes of alcohol can cause a marked elevation of triglyceride levels by stimulating the production of VLDL-triglycerides by the liver (Fig. 3.32).

GOALS FOR DIETARY THERAPY

The first step in treatment of high serum cholesterol, or other forms of dyslipidemia, is dietary therapy. In general, all people over age two should follow an eating plan that will maintain a relatively low level of serum cholesterol and thereby retard the development of atherosclerosis; however, special attention should be given to those who have high serum cholesterol or who are deemed to be at increased risk for CHD. Specifically, a "high-risk" status is conferred on an individual who has an LDL-cholesterol concentration exceeding 160 mg/dl or who has an LDL-cholesterol level in the range of 130 to 159 mg/dl and two other CHD risk factors (see Fig. 2.7). Such individuals should enter active medical therapy for LDL lowering, the first step of which is dietary therapy.

For those who do not fall into the high-risk category, the physician still has a responsibility, although the management and follow-up of these individuals need not be as intensive as with high-risk patients. Individuals whose total cholesterol levels are in the borderline-high zone (200 to 239 mg/dl) and who do not have two other risk factors should be urged to maintain a cholesterol-lowering diet and rechecked on a yearly basis to determine whether their cholesterol levels have fallen to the desirable range. Some authorities believe that the initial classification and the follow-up of these patients are facilitated by measurement of a lipoprotein profile. In general, this decision should be individualized depending on a clinical evaluation of a patient's overall risk status. Particular attention should be given to young adults with borderline-high serum cholesterol, since, owing to the normal rise of cholesterol with age (see Fig. 2.4), they are likely to develop high-risk LDL-cholesterol concentrations later in life and, consequently, must be followed carefully through the years.

The cholesterol-lowering diet to be recommended to those with a borderline-high cholesterol level is the same as the first step of dietary therapy for high-risk patients; however, follow-up is not required for the former as for the latter. Likewise, it is prudent even for those with a desirable serum cholesterol level (less than 200 mg/dl) to adhere to the same diet, but follow-up measurements of total cholesterol in this category of individuals are required only every five years.

For high-risk patients, the ideal goal of therapy is to reduce the LDL-cholesterol level to the desirable range, i.e., below 130 mg/dl. However, the intensity of therapy to be employed can be modified to some extent, depending on the presence or absence of other CHD risk factors. Thus, if one has one or no other risk factors, it may be sufficient to allow the LDL-cholesterol concentration to fall to less than 160 mg/dl, particularly if further lowering would require drug therapy. On the other hand, if two or more risk factors are present, maximal reduction of LDL-cholesterol to below 130 mg/dl is desirable.

In patients with severely elevated levels of total cholesterol (over 325 mg/dl) and LDL-cholesterol (over 220 mg/dl), such as those with heterozygous familial hypercholesterolemia, it is justifiable to turn to drug therapy once persistent severe hypercholesterolemia has been clearly documented. However, these patients are relatively rare, and for most people with more moderate elevations of LDL-cho-

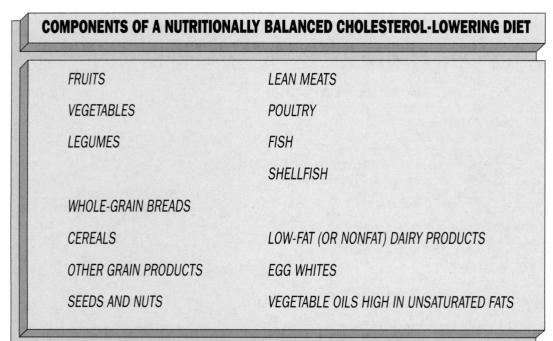

COMPONENTS OF A NUTRITIONALLY BALANCED CHOLESTEROL-LOWERING DIET

FRUITS	LEAN MEATS
VEGETABLES	POULTRY
LEGUMES	FISH
	SHELLFISH
WHOLE-GRAIN BREADS	
CEREALS	LOW-FAT (OR NONFAT) DAIRY PRODUCTS
OTHER GRAIN PRODUCTS	EGG WHITES
SEEDS AND NUTS	VEGETABLE OILS HIGH IN UNSATURATED FATS

Fig. 3.33 Components of a nutritionally balanced cholesterol-lowering diet.

STEP-ONE DIET

NUTRIENT	RECOMMENDATIONS (% of total calories)
Total fat	≤ 30%
Saturated fatty acids	< 10%
Polyunsaturated fatty acids	≤ 10%
Monounsaturated fatty acids	10%–15%
Carbohydrates	50%–60%
Protein	15%

Total calories ⟶	To achieve desirable weight
Cholesterol ⟶	< 300 mg/day

Fig. 3.34 Composition of the Step-One Diet.

lesterol, a prolonged period of dietary therapy is justified before resorting to drug therapy. For monitoring the response to dietary therapy, measurement of LDL-cholesterol is particularly helpful; but if a prolonged period of dietary modification is required, the total cholesterol level can be used as a surrogate for LDL-cholesterol at least on some follow-up determinations.

STEPS OF DIETARY THERAPY
STEP-ONE DIET

The first step of dietary therapy calls for a reduction in intakes of the major and obvious sources of saturated fatty acids and cholesterol, as well as weight reduction to achieve a desirable body weight. Of course, any therapeutic diet should be nutritionally adequate; i.e., it must contain enough protein, vitamins, and minerals to meet the daily requirements. This is best achieved by eating a variety of foods, and the desirable diet should contain fruits, vegetables, legumes (peas and beans), whole-grain and enriched breads, other grains, poultry, fish, lean meat, nonfat and low-fat milk products, egg whites, nuts, and vegetable oils high in unsaturated fats (Fig. 3.33). If such a diet is followed, there will be no danger of malnutrition and enough variety for the diet to be highly palatable.

Recommended Diet. The recommended composition of the Step-One Diet is presented in Figure 3.34. The total fat intake should be approximately 30% of calories. Some authorities believe that the desirable intake of total fat should be below 30% of total calories, whereas others would allow it to be as high as 35% provided that the additional amount is derived from unsaturated fatty acids. Certainly, the intake of saturated fatty acids should be less than 10% of total calories, and for the cholesterol-raising variety of saturates (lauric acid, myristic acid, and palmitic acid), this generally would mean an intake of about 7%. Polyunsaturated fatty acids can be increased up to 10% of total calories as a partial replacement of saturated fatty acids, but many workers believe that polyunsaturates should not exceed 7% of total calories because of possible long-term side effects of high intakes. Monounsaturates will contribute between 10% and 15% of total calories if fat intake is restricted to less than 30%, but the contribution of monounsaturates may rise to as high as 20% of total calories if up to 35% of calories are taken as fat. Carbohydrates will range between 50% and 60% of total calories, whereas protein should not exceed 15% of calories. Cholesterol intake needs to be limited to less than 300 mg/day. Total caloric intake should be reduced to achieve a desirable body weight.

Expected Response. The response to the Step-One Diet will depend on several factors. One is the diet of the patient at the time of entrance to active medical therapy. Because of increased awareness about the dangers of high cholesterol, many people have already modified their diets, and some essentially will be consuming a Step-One Diet at the outset. In these people, a further reduction in cholesterol levels cannot be expected. Furthermore, the inherent responsiveness of people to dietary modification appears to be variable. Some appear to be extremely sensitive to diet, and they will demonstrate a marked reduction in cholesterol levels upon dietary modification. Others are relatively resistant to dietary change, and they may show little decrease in cholesterol levels. The physician must be aware that many individuals with "hypercholesterolemia" on initial screening will demonstrate a response called "regression toward the mean," and on subsequent measurements their cholesterol levels fall to near the mean for the population. This response often is misinterpreted as meaning that a person is highly sensitive to dietary (or drug) therapy when in fact he or she does not have true hypercholesterolemia. For most people who change from a "typical" American diet to the Step-One Diet, a fall in LDL-cholesterol of 20 to 30 mg/dl can be expected. However, some patients who appear to be excessively sensitive to diet will show greater reductions. This is especially the case if they lose weight in addition to modifying the composition of their diet.

Several dietary changes can be made to reduce intakes of saturated fatty acids and cholesterol. If these changes occur, the dietary targets of the Step-One Diet will be achieved. One of the major sources of saturated fatty acids are fatty meats—fatty cuts of beef, pork, and lamb, as well as processed meats (sausage, hot dogs, and bacon); these should be replaced by lean cuts of meat, poultry without skin, and fish (Fig. 3.35). A second source of saturates is whole-milk products—4% fat milk, natural cheeses, ice cream, cream, and whole-milk forms of yogurt and cottage cheese—all of which should be replaced with skim-milk or low-fat (1% or 2% fat) products (Fig. 3.36). Foods that contain "hidden fats" should be decreased. Included in this

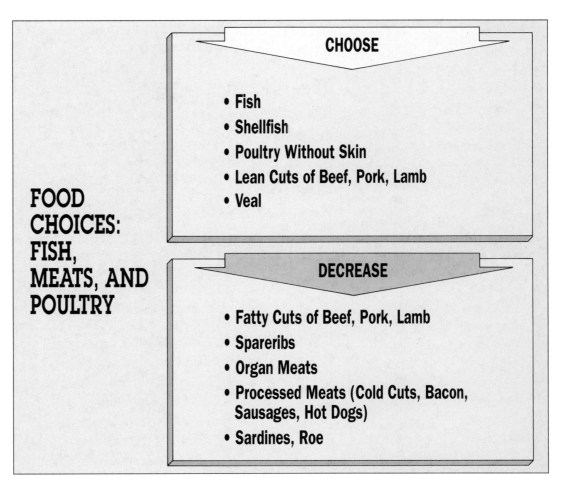

FOOD CHOICES: FISH, MEATS, AND POULTRY

CHOOSE
- Fish
- Shellfish
- Poultry Without Skin
- Lean Cuts of Beef, Pork, Lamb
- Veal

DECREASE
- Fatty Cuts of Beef, Pork, Lamb
- Spareribs
- Organ Meats
- Processed Meats (Cold Cuts, Bacon, Sausages, Hot Dogs)
- Sardines, Roe

Fig. 3.35 Food choices for reducing intakes of saturated fatty acids and cholesterol: fish, meats, and poultry.

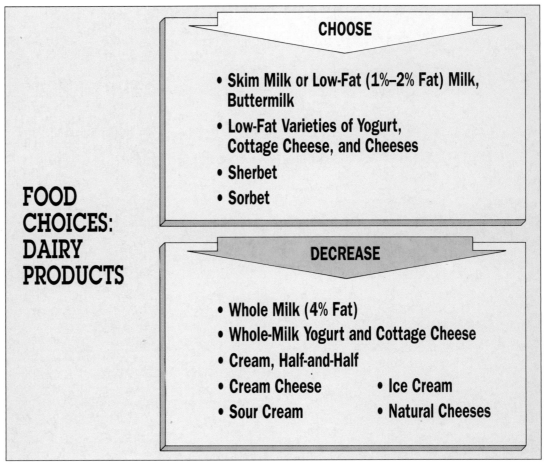

FOOD CHOICES: DAIRY PRODUCTS

CHOOSE
- Skim Milk or Low-Fat (1%–2% Fat) Milk, Buttermilk
- Low-Fat Varieties of Yogurt, Cottage Cheese, and Cheeses
- Sherbet
- Sorbet

DECREASE
- Whole Milk (4% Fat)
- Whole-Milk Yogurt and Cottage Cheese
- Cream, Half-and-Half
- Cream Cheese
- Sour Cream
- Ice Cream
- Natural Cheeses

Fig. 3.36 Food choices for reducing intakes of saturated fatty acids and cholesterol: dairy products.

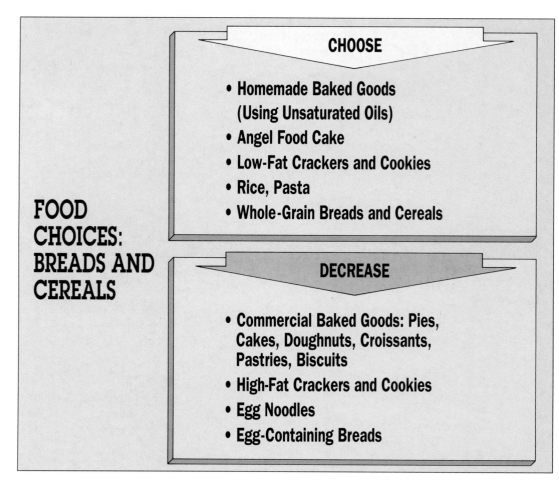

Fig. 3.37 Food choices for reducing intakes of saturated fatty acids and cholesterol: breads and cereals.

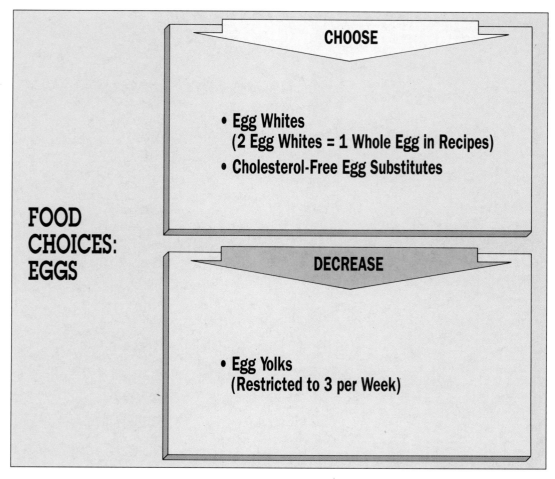

Fig. 3.38 Food choices for reducing intakes of cholesterol: eggs.

category are many commercial baked goods (e.g., pies, cakes, doughnuts, croissants, pastries, muffins, biscuits, and high-fat crackers and cookies). Hidden sources of cholesterol are egg noodles and breads in which eggs are an ingredient. These commercial baked goods should be replaced by home-made products that minimize use of saturated oils, as well as by angel food cake, low-fat crackers and cookies, rice, pasta, and whole-grain breads (Fig. 3.37).

Where possible, egg yolks should be replaced with egg whites or cholesterol-free egg substitutes (Fig. 3.38). In many recipes, two egg whites can be used for one whole egg. In general, to meet the recommended intake for cholesterol, egg yolks should be restricted to about three per week. Fruits and vegetables are desirable; however, fruit should not be covered with cream or ice cream, and vegetables should be prepared without butter, cream, or other sauces (Fig. 3.39). When oils are used for cooking or for dressings, unsaturated oils are preferable to saturated fats (Fig. 3.40). The oils can be high in either monoun-saturates (olive oil, canola oil) or poly-unsaturates (corn oil, safflower oil, soy-bean oil, or sunflower oil). Margarines made from vegetables should be used instead of butter as a spread. Shorten-ings prepared from vegetable oils are to be chosen in the place of those hav-ing lard or large amounts of tropical oils (palm oil, palm kernel oil, or coconut oil). Other sources of unsaturated oils are most seeds and nuts and several brands of mayonnaise and salad dress-ings. Fortunately, it is becoming easier to make these changes. The food indus-try is responding with the development of new foods products low in total fat, saturated fatty acids, and cholesterol that can be used in the place of cholesterol-raising foods.

Role of Physician and Staff. The first step of dietary therapy is more than just a recommended composition of the diet. It is an approach to the control of high serum cholesterol within the physician's office. The physician and immediate staff should develop the expertise and back-up educational materials required to carry out this first step of therapy. The knowledge and attitude of the physician largely determine the success of dietary therapy. If the physician takes a positive and optimistic attitude, the patient is more likely to respond in kind and to show an adequate cholesterol lowering without the need for drug therapy. The physician should take the time required to explain the nature of the cholesterol problem and to outline the general approach to therapy. Within the constraints of available time, a dietary history should be taken, and points requiring modification to meet the aims of the Step-One Diet explained. Finally, the physician plays a vital role in monitoring the response to dietary modification. The physician's message can be reinforced by the immediate staff, particularly registered nurses, registered physician's assistants, nurse clinicians, and other types of assistants. These individuals should take the opportunity to attend training courses on instruction in dietary modification, and they should obtain essential educational materials for the patient. In general, it is not necessary to turn to registered dietitians for the first step of diet modification. Indeed, a majority of patients with high serum cholesterol should respond

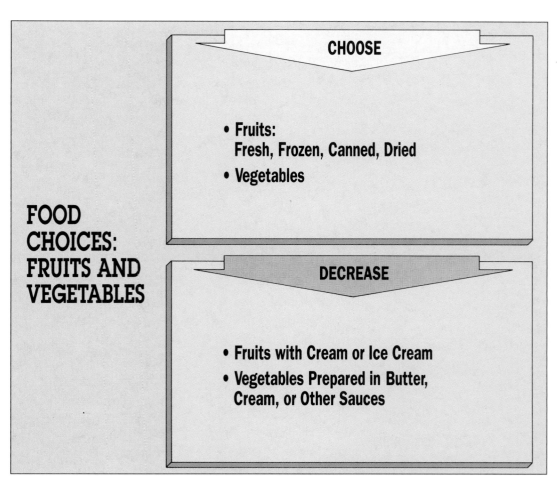

Fig. 3.39 Food choices for reducing intakes of saturated fatty acids and cholesterol: fruits and vegetables.

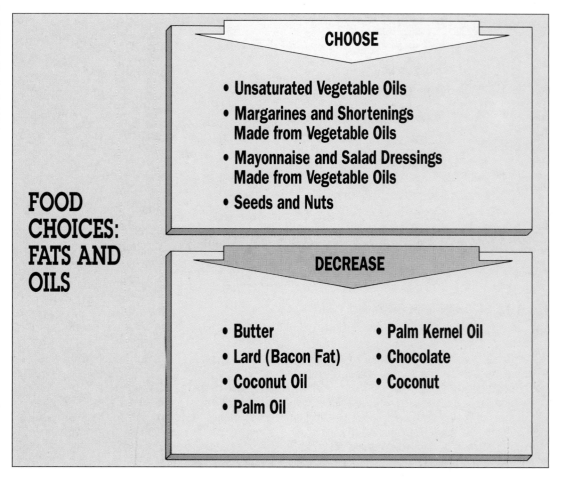

Fig. 3.40 Food choices for reducing intakes of saturated fatty acids and cholesterol: fats and oils.

STEP-ONE DIET FOLLOW-UP

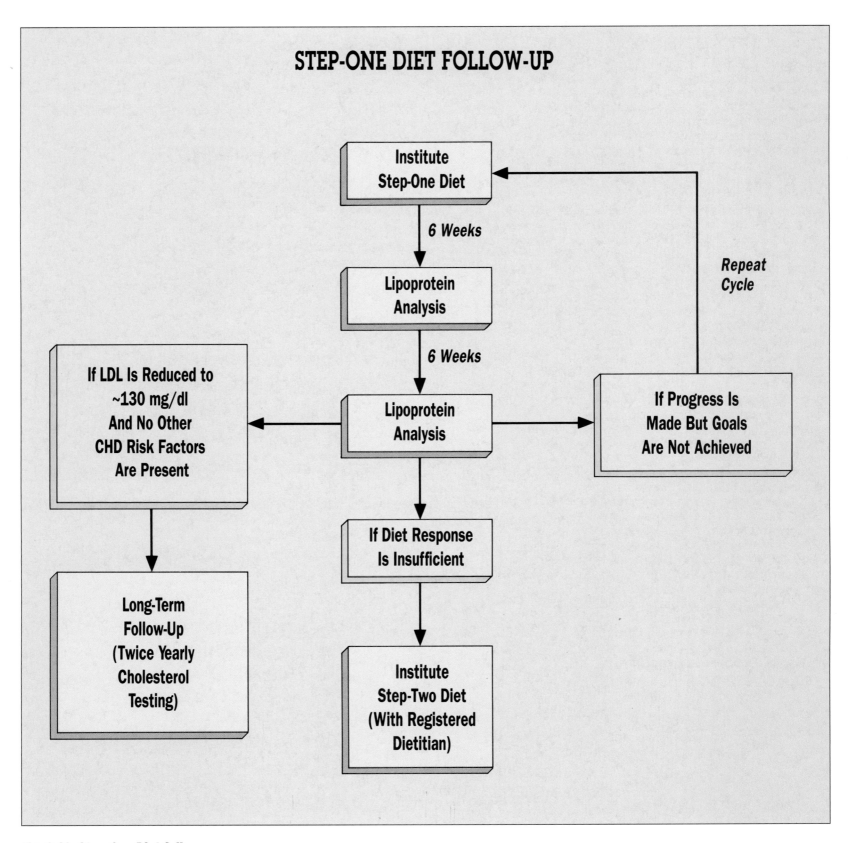

Fig. 3.41 Step-One Diet follow-up.

adequately to the Step-One Diet without the need for more extensive dietary modification or drug therapy.

Follow-up Schedule. The Step-One Diet should be continued for a period of at least three months before consideration of more intensive dietary therapy (Fig. 3.41). Repeat measurements of lipoproteins should be carried out at six weeks and three months. If progress is being made but the goals of therapy have not been achieved during this period, it may be appropriate to extend the Step-One Diet for another three months. Most patients require considerable time to learn new dietary habits, and if progress is being made, more time should be allowed. Moreover, several months may be needed for the weight reduction advocated by the Step-One Diet. For most patients, weight reduction is just as important as, if not more important than, change in diet composition for reducing the LDL-cholesterol level and for producing a favorable overall change in the lipoprotein profile. If despite thorough follow-up in the physician's office, the goals of LDL-lowering therapy are not achieved, consideration must be given to going to the Step-Two Diet, which, as discussed below, usually requires involvement of a registered dietitian.

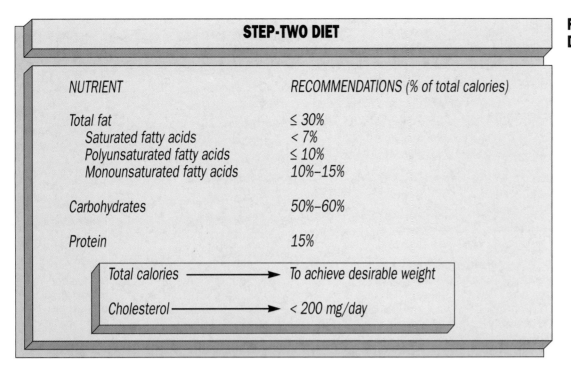

STEP-TWO DIET

NUTRIENT	RECOMMENDATIONS (% of total calories)
Total fat	≤ 30%
Saturated fatty acids	< 7%
Polyunsaturated fatty acids	≤ 10%
Monounsaturated fatty acids	10%–15%
Carbohydrates	50%–60%
Protein	15%

Total calories ⟶ To achieve desirable weight

Cholesterol ⟶ < 200 mg/day

Fig. 3.42 Composition of the Step-Two Diet.

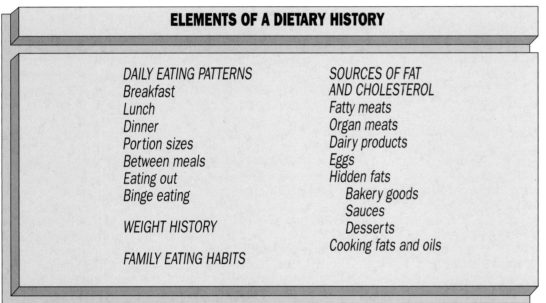

ELEMENTS OF A DIETARY HISTORY

DAILY EATING PATTERNS
Breakfast
Lunch
Dinner
Portion sizes
Between meals
Eating out
Binge eating

WEIGHT HISTORY

FAMILY EATING HABITS

SOURCES OF FAT
AND CHOLESTEROL
Fatty meats
Organ meats
Dairy products
Eggs
Hidden fats
    Bakery goods
    Sauces
    Desserts
Cooking fats and oils

Fig. 3.43 Elements of a dietary history.

Finally, if the LDL-cholesterol concentration approaches 130 mg/dl, particularly if other risk factors are present, long-term follow-up is required. Total cholesterol measurements should be made twice a year to confirm adherence to the diet and to reinforce dietary and behavior modification.

STEP-TWO DIET

The second step of dietary therapy represents an attempt to intensify management of elevated LDL-cholesterol to meet the goals of therapy without the necessity of turning to drug therapy. The essence of the Step-Two Diet is the utilization of a registered dietitian to assist the patient in making the dietary modifications necessary to achieve the goals of therapy. In addition, this diet calls for further dietary restrictions as one means to achieve the therapeutic goal. However, the Step-Two Diet, car-

ried out under the supervision of a registered dietitian, requires more than further dietary restrictions. It makes use of assessment of nutritional status and eating habits, nutrition education, behavior modification, monitoring and reinforcement, and involvement of the family in dietary therapy. Although these same principles should be used in the physician's office, they are best carried out with the assistance of a registered dietitian.

Recommended Diet. With the Step-Two Diet, the intake of total fat remains at 30% or less of total calories, but saturated fatty acids should be reduced to below 7% of total calories (as opposed to less than 10% in the Step-One Diet) and cholesterol intake to less than 200 mg/day (300 mg/day in the Step-One Diet) (Fig. 3.42). Intakes of polyunsaturated and monounsaturated fatty acids are maintained at the Step-One level, as are carbohydrates and protein. If

the patient is overweight, efforts to achieve a desirable body weight should be redoubled.

Role of Registered Dietitian. The registered dietitian is the key element to the success of the Step-Two Diet. Registered dietitians are trained in the principles of clinical nutrition and in dietary intervention. The physician can find a registered dietitian through the American Dietetic Association (208 South LaSalle Street, Chicago, Illinois 60604), from dietetic departments of most large hospitals or schools of allied health, or the local affiliate of the American Heart Association. Many dietitians are presently gaining the expertise to manage the dietary problems associated with high serum cholesterol.

Dietary History. To plan the Step-Two Diet, the dietitian first takes a detailed history of the patient's eating habits (Fig. 3.43). The daily eating pattern is reviewed. Does the patient eat break-

**Fig. 3.44 Factors responsible for an inade-
quate response to dietary therapy.**

FACTORS RESPONSIBLE FOR INADEQUATE RESPONSE TO DIETARY THERAPY

SEVERE HYPERCHOLESTEROLEMIA

MODERATE HYPERCHOLESTEROLEMIA RESISTANT TO DIETARY MODIFICATION

INABILITY OF PATIENTS TO MODIFY DIET

NEED FOR MORE TIME TO MODIFY DIET

fast, lunch, and dinner every day? Which meals are routinely skipped? What is eaten between meals? Does the patient engage in binge eating? How often does the patient eat out in restaurants or at the work place? What foods are chosen when eating out? The family's eating pattern is also reviewed. A weight history is recorded particularly if the patient is overweight. Of most importance, the dietitian attempts to discern the sources of total fat, saturated fatty acids, cholesterol, and excess calories in the patient's diet.

Instruction and Behavior Modification. On the basis of the dietary history, the dietitian provides essential instruction on dietary modification. It may be necessary for the patient to relearn the recommendations and principles of the Step-One Diet before advancing to those of the Step-Two Diet. The basic connection between the diet and high serum cholesterol levels is discussed. The concept that three major dietary components—saturated fatty acids, cholesterol, and excess total calories—are the primary causes of elevated serum cholesterol is reemphasized. The sources of these cholesterol-raising factors in the diet, and substitutes that will not raise cholesterol levels, are reviewed. Moreover, methods for measurement of portion sizes and food weights are taught.

Sessions with the dietitian will emphasize practical aspects of dietary modifications. Attention should be given to the problems of eating out, occasional dietary splurges, making substitutions of desirable foods for undesirable ones, involvement with family eating habits, difficulties with weight reduction, and feelings of failure in diet modification.

For obese individuals, the principles of behavior modification should be employed. This approach gives the best chance for long-term weight reduction. Failure to lose weight in obese persons is one of the major causes for diet failure in patients with hypercholesterolemia.

Involvement of the family in dietary change usually is necessary for the success of dietary therapy in an individual. If one eats most meals at home, it is necessary for the person who prepares the meals to be committed to dietary change. Since high cholesterol levels tend to run in families, there are medical as well as social reasons for "treating" the whole family.

For interaction with a registered dietitian to be successful, it will be necessary for many patients to have a long-term relationship with the dietitian. One or two instructional sessions usually are not enough. Dietary change is a slow process, and unless there is a permanent change in eating behavior, dietary therapy will not be successful. Many people must remain involved with both a physician and a dietitian before long-term success can be assured. Continued education and reinforcement usually are necessary.

Finally, the importance of exercise for successful dietary therapy should not be overlooked. Exercise burns off excess calories and saturated fatty acids. Therefore, it helps to lower the LDL-cholesterol level in conjunction with overall dietary modification. The action of regular and vigorous exercise to lower the triglyceride concentration and to raise HDL-cholesterol is well known. Therefore, the patient should be encouraged to begin an exercise program that is appropriate for his or her general health.

Expected Response. In general, the Step-Two Diet should give a better LDL-lowering response than the Step-One Diet. Not only will the patient benefit from the intensive therapy of a registered dietitian, but the Step-Two Diet has a lower content of both saturated fatty acids and cholesterol. Actually, a greater benefit is likely to accrue from better adherence to a cholesterol-lowering diet than from further diet modification. From the latter, an additional fall in LDL-cholesterol levels of 10 to 15 mg/dl can be expected, provided a modification in the diet actually is made.

Follow-up Schedule. The follow-up of the patient on the Step-Two Diet is similar to that on the Step-One Diet (see Fig. 3.41). Lipoprotein analysis should be carried out at six weeks and three months. If progress is being made, but the individual has not reached an LDL-cholesterol level of between 130 and 160 mg/dl, or preferably lower, a repeat cycle of the Step-Two Diet is in order. If the goal for LDL lowering is reached, long-term monitoring and reinforcement are necessary. However, if the patient's LDL-cholesterol level remains unacceptably high in spite of an adequate trial on the Step-Two Diet, consideration will have to be given to drug therapy (see Unit Four).

Several factors may be responsible for an inadequate response to dietary therapy (Fig. 3.44). First, if patients have severe forms of hypercholesterolemia, dietary therapy alone usually will not be sufficient to reduce the LDL-cholesterol levels to an acceptable range; in such patients, drug therapy is justified without a prolonged trial of dietary treatment. Second, some patients with only moderate hypercholesterolemia are relatively resistant to dietary change and, in spite of adequate diet modification, decrease their LDL-cholesterol levels only a few milligrams per deciliter. Third, some patients cannot successfully modify their diets despite reasonable efforts by the physician and staff. And fourth, there are individuals who are capable of modifying their diets, but more time is needed. These are individuals who need to be "recycled" in their follow-up to dietary therapy as outlined in Figure 3.41.

ROLE OF DIETARY THERAPY IN SPECIAL GROUPS
ELDERLY PATIENTS

Many elderly individuals, both men and women, have elevated LDL-cholesterol levels. There is growing evidence that elevated LDL-cholesterol still contributes to increased coronary risk in the elderly. Consequently, if an older individual is deemed to be in overall good health and has a relatively good long-term prognosis, an attempt at lowering the LDL-cholesterol levels can be justified. However, most of these people are not candidates for lipid-lowering drugs and, therefore, dietary therapy is preferable. Even so, radical modification of the diet should be avoided in older people because of the tendency of many elderly people to eat inadequate diets. Thus, the Step-One Diet is to be preferred to the more restrictive Step-Two Diet. On balance, a slightly elevated LDL-cholesterol in older people is preferable to the development of malnutrition.

PREGNANT WOMEN

Normally, serum cholesterol and triglyceride levels rise during the third trimester of pregnancy. Although triglyceride concentrations usually return to normal within two months after delivery, elevated serum cholesterol may persist for several months. A prolonged period of hypercholesterolemia after delivery may indicate the presence of a genetic form of hyperlipidemia. In the rare instances of women with primary or secondary forms of chylomicronemia, extreme increases in triglyceride concentrations may occur, putting the patients at high risk for acute pancreatitis. A diet very low in fat, i.e., 10% or less of total calories, is required to maintain triglyceride levels in a low-risk range.

HETEROZYGOUS FAMILIAL HYPERCHOLESTEROLEMIA

In patients with this disorder, who have severe elevations of LDL-cholesterol, dietary therapy is rarely sufficient to achieve an acceptable cholesterol level. In such people, drug therapy usually is required. Still, diet modification is a useful adjunct to drug therapy, and a heterozygous hypercholesterolemic patient should be taught the principles of the Step-Two Diet. However, it is not necessary to complete the adjustment to diet modification before resorting to drug therapy.

MODERATE TO SEVERE PRIMARY HYPERCHOLESTEROLEMIA

Many hypercholesterolemic patients present with marked elevations of LDL-cholesterol (above 200 to 220 mg/dl) without clinical evidence of heterozygous familial hypercholesterolemia (e.g., strong family history of high cholesterol and tendon xanthomas). Even so, these patients can be treated in a similar way to those with familial hypercholesterolemia. Their serum LDL-cholesterol levels frequently cannot be brought to a desirable level by diet alone, and drug treatment is required. Like patients with familial hypercholesterolemia, it is not necessary to continue dietary therapy alone for a prolonged period before turning to drug therapy. Once it becomes apparent that the LDL level cannot be brought down satisfactorily by diet alone, drug treatment can be started. For patients with more moderate elevations of LDL-cholesterol (160 to 200 mg/dl), intensive dietary therapy, as described in this unit, should be carried out before turning to drug therapy.

FAMILIAL DYSBETALIPOPROTEINEMIA (TYPE III HLP)

Many patients with type III HLP are overweight, and in these patients, weight reduction frequently normalizes their serum lipid levels. Some patients with type III HLP have diabetes mellitus, and control of hyperglycemia and weight reduction produce a marked improvement in their lipoprotein pattern. If plasma lipid levels in type III HLP patients cannot be normalized by diet modification alone, it may be necessary to employ lipid-lowering drug therapy. (See Unit Two, pp 2.11–2.12 and Fig. 2.19.)

SEVERE HYPERTRIGLYCERIDEMIA

If a patient has severe elevations of triglycerides with either type I HLP (see Fig. 2.17) or type V HLP (see Fig. 2.21), marked restriction of dietary fat is required to reduce concentrations of chylomicrons so as to decrease the risk for acute pancreatitis. The percentage of dietary fat must be reduced to less than 15% of total calories, and sometimes even further. The diet can be made more palatable for some patients by the use of medium-chain triglycerides, which are not incorporated into chylomicrons. In the absence of lipoprotein lipase (type I HLP), diet modification is the only effective mode of therapy. For those with type V HLP, weight reduction and better control of hyperglycemia (if diabetes mellitus is present) help decrease the severity of chylomicronemia. If diet modification proves ineffective in treatment of chylomicronemia, drug treatment may be required (see Unit Four).

HYPOALPHALIPOPROTEINEMIA

In most patients with low HDL-cholesterol levels, the decrease in HDL is due to environmental and hygienic causes (see Fig. 2.10). Cigarette smoking is one cause, and the HDL level is further reduced by concomitant heavy intake of coffee. The smoker, therefore, should be urged to stop smoking and/or to reduce excess coffee intake. Both weight reduction in obese patients and increased exercise will raise HDL-cholesterol levels. Weight reduction raises HDL levels both by mitigating hypertriglyceridemia and by decreasing stores of adipose tissue. Anabolic steroids can cause profound reduction in HDL-cholesterol levels, and their use should be strongly discouraged in young adults.

DIABETIC DYSLIPIDEMIA

The dyslipidemia of diabetic patients (see Fig. 2.40) can be improved by weight reduction if the patient is obese, and by better control of hyperglycemia. These beneficial effects can be potentiated by starting an exercise program and reducing consumption of alcohol.

Unit Four

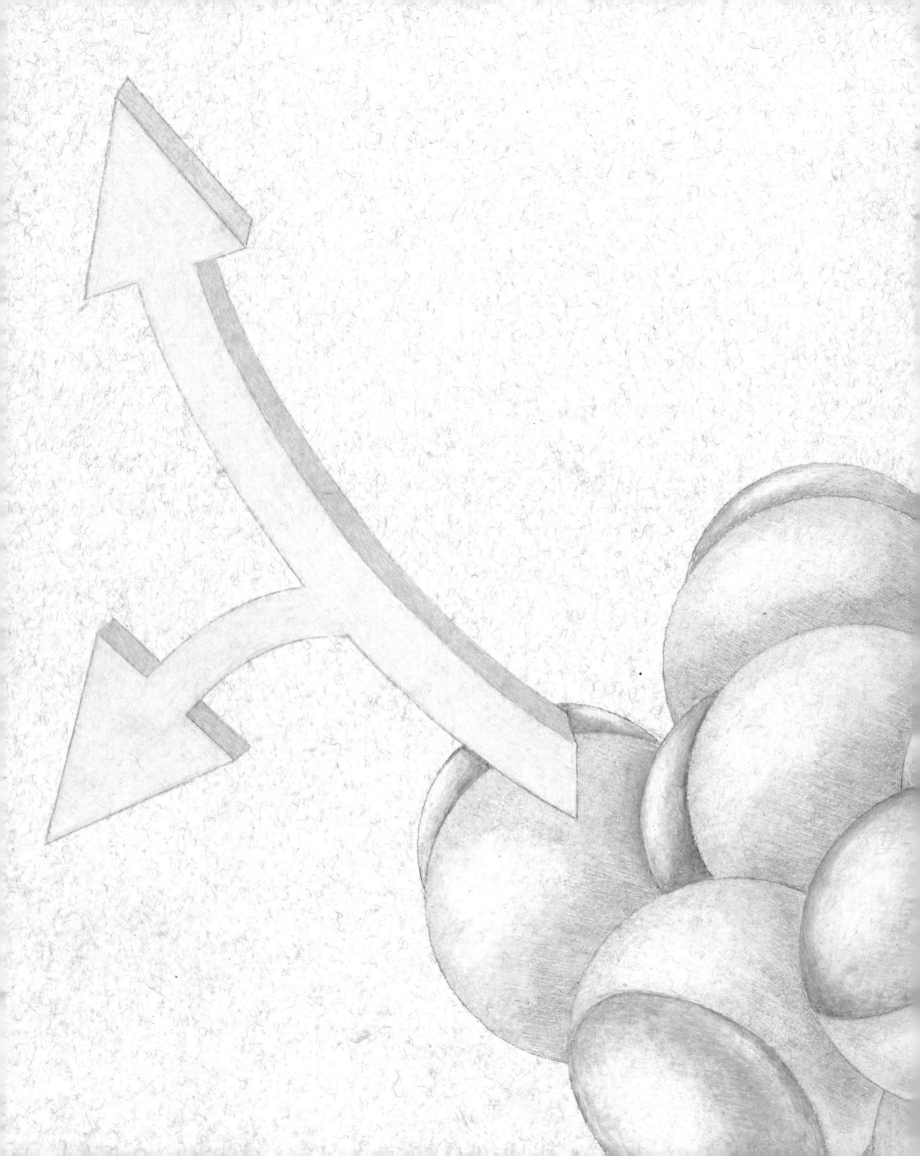

DRUG THERAPY OF HYPERLIPIDEMIA

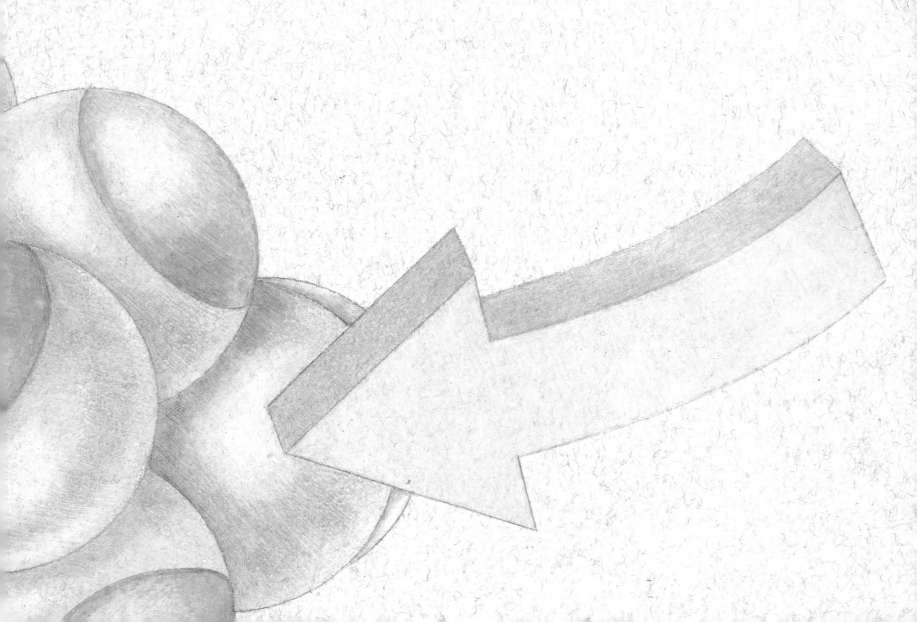

In the past decade, major advances have been made in the treatment of hyperlipidemia with drugs. New drugs have been developed that are highly effective for lowering serum lipid levels, and the potential usefulness and indications of older drugs have been better defined. Efficacy in reduction of risk for coronary heart disease (CHD) has been demonstrated for several drugs, and their side-effect profiles have been described. The action of drugs to produce additive responses when used in combination now makes possible the "normalization" of serum lipid levels in most patients, even in those with severe hyperlipidemia. This unit is concerned with the indications and goals for drug therapy, the choice of drugs (including their structures, mechanisms of action, efficacy and specific indications), and their use in combination with other drugs.

INDICATIONS FOR DRUG THERAPY

A critical question in the management of hyperlipidemia is when to use lipid-lowering drugs. General guidelines for use of drugs are outlined in Figure 4.1. For patients with hyperlipidemia, dietary modification is the first line of treatment, and for most patients, a prolonged trial of dietary therapy is indicated (see Unit Three) before resorting to drug treatment. If a patient has severe hyperlipidemia, it may be justifiable to begin dietary and drug therapy simultaneously. This latter approach is appropriate for patients with severe hypercholesterolemia, especially heterozygous familial hypercholesterolemia (FH), and severe chylomicromia (type V hyperlipoproteinemia). The second major indication for drug therapy is moderate hypercholesterolemia in which dietary therapy has failed to produce a satisfactory reduction in cholesterol levels. As a general rule, patients with moderate hypercholesterolemia who are at high risk for CHD from other causes are better candidates for drug therapy than those at low risk.

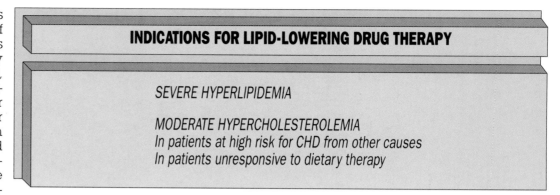

INDICATIONS FOR LIPID-LOWERING DRUG THERAPY

SEVERE HYPERLIPIDEMIA

MODERATE HYPERCHOLESTEROLEMIA
In patients at high risk for CHD from other causes
In patients unresponsive to dietary therapy

Fig. 4.1 Indications for lipid-lowering drug therapy.

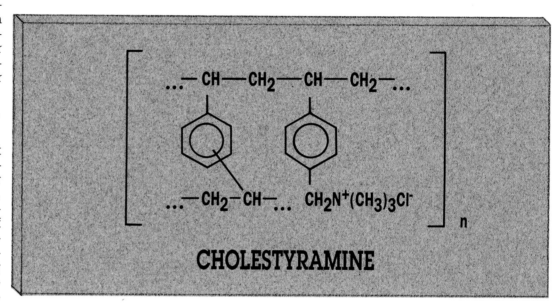

Fig. 4.2 Structural formula of cholestyramine.

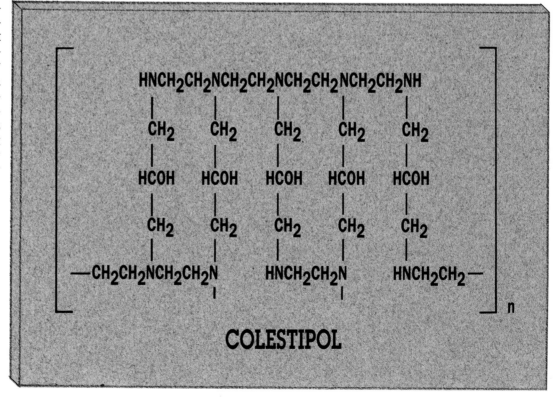

Fig. 4.3 Structural formula of colestipol.

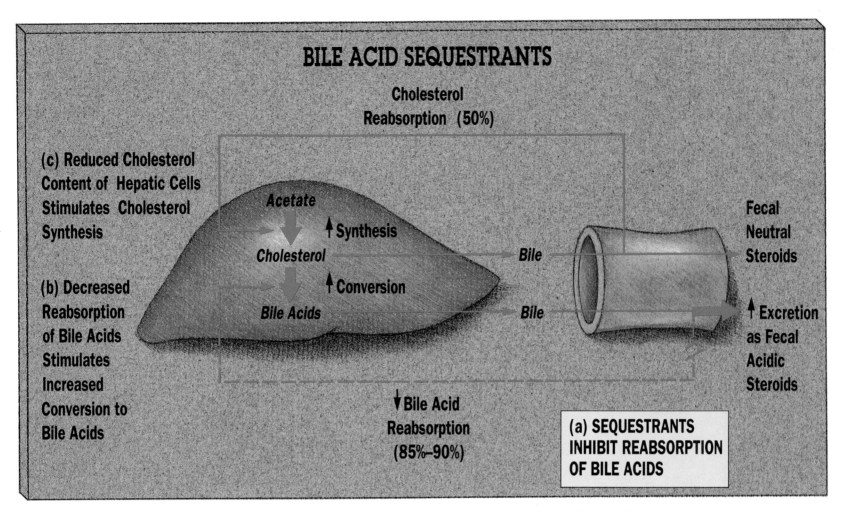

Fig. 4.4 Site of action of the bile acid sequestrants and their effects on bile-acid and cholesterol metabolism.

BILE ACID SEQUESTRANTS

The bile acid sequestrants are resins that bind bile acids in the intestinal tract and enhance their excretion in stools. The production of bile acids from cholesterol causes a drain on hepatic stores of cholesterol, leading ultimately to a reduction of serum LDL-cholesterol levels. The bile acid sequestrants have been proven to be effective for reducing risk for CHD, and they generally are safe. Because of long-term experience with these drugs, their proven safety, and their demonstrated efficacy for decreasing CHD risk, the bile acid sequestrants are considered first-line drugs for treatment of hypercholesterolemia.

AVAILABLE DRUGS

Two bile acid sequestrants are available for treatment of hypercholesterolemia, cholestyramine and colestipol (Figs. 4.2, 4.3). Both are quaternary amines with multiple positive charges

that bind to negatively charged bile acids in the intestinal tract. Since neither cholestyramine nor colestipol is absorbed in its passage through the gut, their action on serum cholesterol levels is entirely secondary to their effects within the intestinal lumen. Not only do the sequestrants bind bile acids, but they bind to other negatively charged ions, including some drugs. This latter effect must be taken into consideration when a bile acid sequestrant is used with other drugs.

MECHANISMS OF ACTION

Effects on Bile-Acid and Cholesterol Metabolism. The bile acid sequestrants bind to bile acids in the small intestine and partially prevent their absorption (Fig. 4.4). Normally, approximately 97% to 98% of all bile acids entering the intestine are reabsorbed in the ileum. Bile acids return to the liver through the portal vein and are cleared almost completely in their first pass through the liver. They

are rapidly resecreted into bile to complete the enterohepatic circulation (see Fig. 1.6). In the liver, the bile acids inhibit the conversion of cholesterol into bile acids by feedback inhibition. During therapy with bile acid sequestrants, reabsorption of bile acids is decreased to 85% to 90%. This reduces the flux of bile acids back to the liver, thereby releasing feedback inhibition on conversion of cholesterol into bile acids. As more cholesterol is transformed into bile acids, the hepatic content of cholesterol falls. One response to this change is a compensatory increase in the synthesis of cholesterol, a change that occurs for the purpose of restoring the balance of cholesterol within liver cells. (See also the discussion on "Cholesterol Metabolism" in Unit One, pp 1.2–1.6.)

Actions on Lipoprotein Metabolism. The action of bile acid sequestrants in reducing the cholesterol content of liver cells enhances transcription of the gene encoding for LDL receptors; the result is an increase in the number of

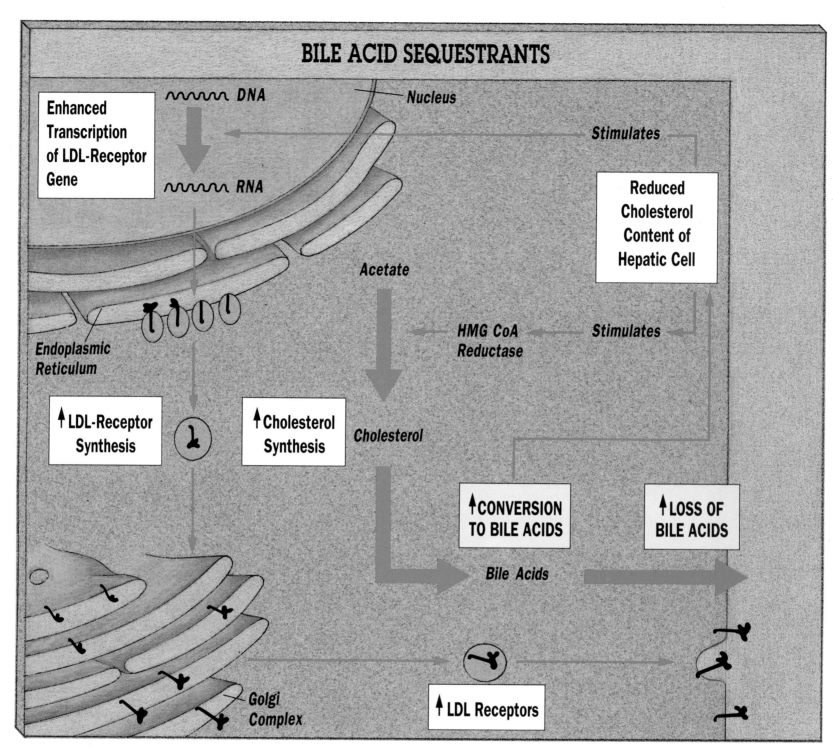

Fig. 4.5 Effects of reduced cholesterol content of hepatic cells, secondary to the actions of bile acid sequestrants, on the synthesis of cholesterol and LDL receptors.

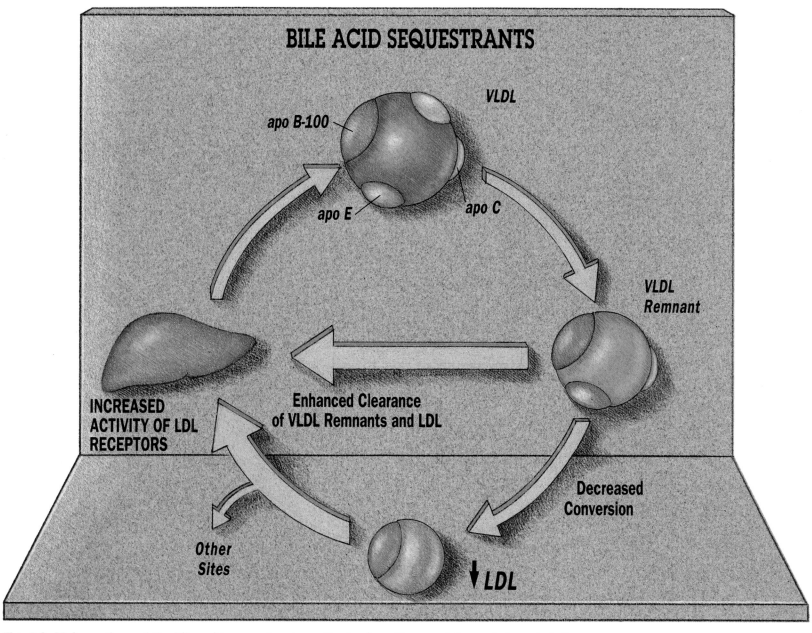

Fig. 4.6 Major actions of the bile acid sequestrants on the basic pathways of lipoprotein metabolism.

LDL receptors on the surface of liver cells (Fig. 4.5). The resulting rise in LDL-receptor activity has two effects on lipoprotein metabolism. First, it increases the clearance of LDL, which tends to lower the LDL-cholesterol concentration; and second, it promotes the clearance of VLDL and VLDL remnants, which decreases conversion of VLDL to LDL (Fig. 4.6). The latter effect further reduces concentrations of LDL-cholesterol. Decreases in LDL-cholesterol levels in the range of 15% to 25% are typical with bile acid sequestrants, but some patients obtain even greater responses.

In many individuals, therapy with bile acid sequestrants may cause a modest increase in HDL-cholesterol levels; the average increase is only about 2 to 4 mg/dl, but occasional patients show an even greater rise. The mechanism for the increase in HDL levels with sequestrant therapy is unknown.

Another action of bile acid sequestrants is to raise serum concentrations of VLDL-triglycerides. The cause of this response is an enhanced secretion of VLDL-triglycerides by the liver. The reason why bile acid sequestrants promote hepatic synthesis of VLDL-triglycerides has not been determined. In patients

with mild hypertriglyceridemia, sequestrants can cause a striking increase in triglyceride levels. For patients with marked hypertriglyceridemia, bile acid sequestrants are contraindicated. In the latter patients, sequestrant therapy can greatly accentuate elevations in triglyceride concentration and may cause development of acute pancreatitis.

DOSAGE

Both cholestyramine and colestipol are powders that must be dispersed in water or fruit juices before ingestion. Cholestyramine also can be obtained

DOSAGES OF BILE ACID SEQUESTRANTS

| DRUG | DOSE | | |
	LOW	MODERATE	HIGH
Cholestyramine	4 g BID	8 g BID	8 g TID
Colestipol	5 g BID	10 g BID	10 g TID

Fig. 4.7 Dosages of the bile acid sequestrants.

SIDE EFFECTS OF BILE ACID SEQUESTRANTS

GASTROINTESTINAL
Constipation
Epigastric fullness and distress
Abdominal discomfort

LIPID
Rise in serum triglycerides

Fig. 4.8 Side effects of the bile acid sequestrants.

INTERACTION OF BILE ACID SEQUESTRANTS WITH OTHER DRUGS

INTERFERENCE WITH ABSORPTION OF
Digoxin and digitoxin
Warfarin
Thiazide diuretics
Beta-adrenergic blocking agents
Thyroid and thyroxine preparations

Fig. 4.9 Interaction of the bile acid sequestrants with other drugs.

INDICATIONS FOR BILE ACID SEQUESTRANTS

PRIMARY HYPERCHOLESTEROLEMIA
(without concomitant
hypertriglyceridemia)

PRIMARY MIXED HYPERLIPIDEMIA
(in combination with triglyceride-
lowering drugs)

Fig. 4.10 Indications for bile acid sequestrants.

in a more convenient bar form. Four grams of cholestyramine are equivalent to five grams of colestipol for bile acid binding. The drugs usually are given twice daily, but sometimes three times. They can be taken in low, moderate, and high doses (Fig. 4.7). Both effectiveness and side effects increase with increasing dosage. For many patients, low doses are readily tolerated and produce a satisfactory lowering of LDL-cholesterol levels. In other patients, higher doses may be required to obtain the desired response.

SIDE EFFECTS

The bile acid sequestrants have several side effects, which generally are not serious (Fig. 4.8). Their major adverse effects are gastrointestinal; among these, constipation is the most common and usually is worse at higher doses. Additional gastrointestinal side effects include bloating, epigastric fullness, nausea, flatulence, and occasionally even diarrhea. Although sequestrants generally are the drug of first choice for cholesterol lowering, they may not

be tolerated in patients having chronic constipation, hemorrhoids, peptic ulcer disease, or persistent esophageal reflux. Nevertheless, if the drug is started in low doses, it still may be possible to work the dose upward to a therapeutic level even in patients with these complaints. Constipation often can be mitigated by increasing dietary fiber or by stool softeners; laxatives generally should be avoided.

The bile acid sequestrants can interfere with the absorption of other drugs (Fig. 4.9). The most common agents thought to be affected are digitalis products, warfarin, thyroxine, thiazide diuretics, beta-adrenergic blocking agents, and possibly other drugs. To obtain maximal bioavailability of these other drugs, it is advisable for the patient to take them one hour before or four hours after administration of a bile acid sequestrant. High doses of sequestrants may interfere with absorption of fat-soluble vitamins (vitamins A, D, and K) and folic acid, although a definite vitamin deficiency occurring during administration of bile acid sequestrants has not been reported.

In large clinical trials, a few patients taking bile acid sequestrants have shown transitory increases in hepatic transaminases or alkaline phosphatase. It is difficult to visualize a mechanism whereby sequestrant therapy could have adverse effects on liver function, and these changes may be incidental findings. As mentioned before, serum triglycerides can be raised during sequestrant therapy.

INDICATIONS

The indications for use of a bile acid sequestrant are given in Figure 4.10. The major indication is elevation of LDL-cholesterol, particularly when such elevation is an isolated abnormality. Sequestrants are less effective in patients with concomitant hypertriglyceridemia. However, they may be used in patients with mixed hyperlipidemia by combining them with triglyceride-lowering drugs. (See also discussion below on "Primary Mixed Hyperlipidemia.")

Strong evidence for the efficacy and safety of bile acids sequestrants in the

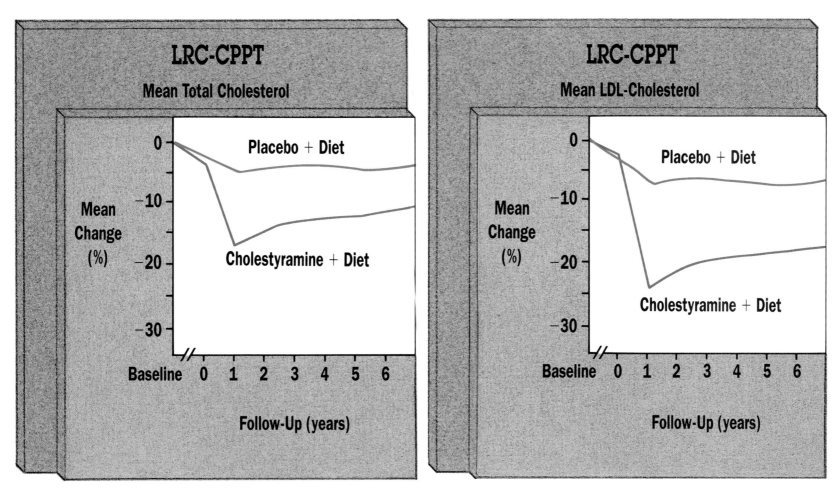

Fig. 4.11 Comparison of reductions in mean total cholesterol (left) and mean LDL-cholesterol (right) in participants observing a cholesterol-lowering diet and receiving either placebo or cholestyramine in the LRC-CPPT study.

treatment of high LDL-cholesterol was obtained in the Lipid Research Clinics Coronary Primary Prevention Trial (LRC-CPPT). This trial recruited 3,806 middle-aged men having LDL-cholesterol levels exceeding 190 mg/dl. The subjects were divided into two groups—placebo and cholestyramine—and all subjects were started on a cholesterol-lowering diet. They continued on placebo or cholestyramine regimens for a minimum of seven years and some up to ten years. Dietary modification caused only a mild reduction in cholesterol levels, whereas cholestyramine therapy induced a 14% decrease in total cholesterol and a 21% lowering of LDL-cholesterol during the first year of trial, as compared with baseline (Fig. 4.11). The number of coronary events in the two experimental groups is presented in Figure 4.12. These events included definite CHD death and nonfatal myocardial infarction. There were 187 events in the placebo group and 155 in the cholestyramine group. The percentage difference of 19% was statistically significant at $p < 0.05$. The difference between the two groups extended to other

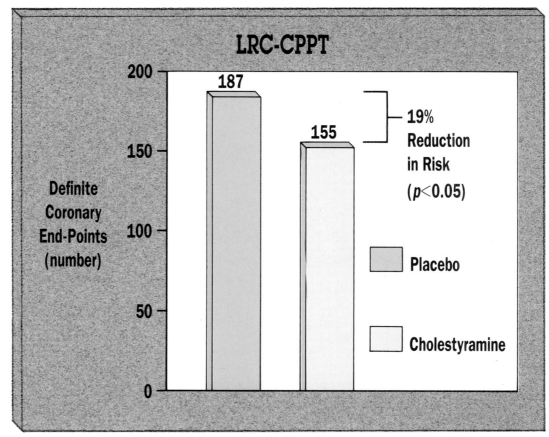

Fig. 4.12 Comparison of the incidence of definite coronary end-points (definite CHD death and nonfatal myocardial infarction) in the cholestyramine and placebo groups in the LRC-CPPT study.

Fig. 4.13 Life-table cumulative incidence of primary end-points in the cholestyramine and placebo groups in the LRC-CPPT study.

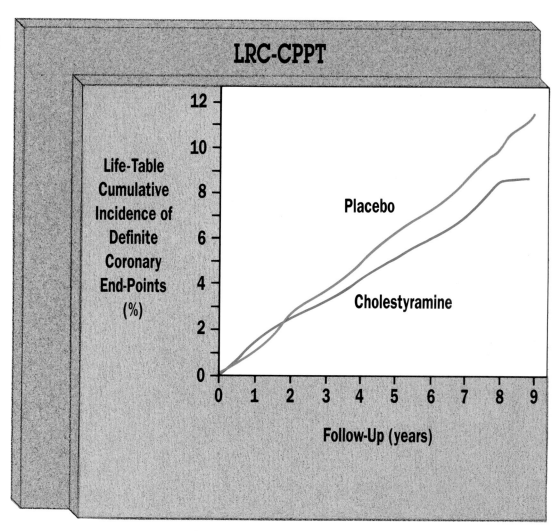

Fig. 4.14 Relationship between the percentage reduction in LDL-cholesterol and the percentage reduction in CHD risk (by the Cox proportional hazards model) for participants in the LRC-CPPT study.

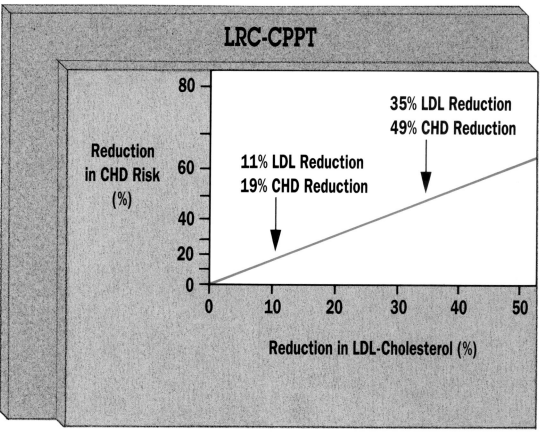

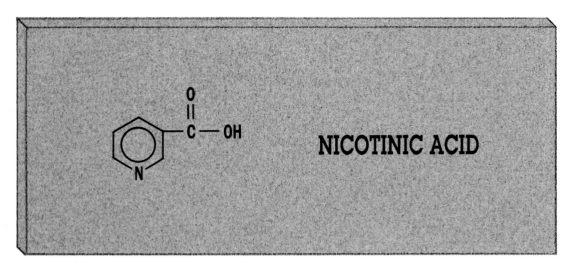

Fig. 4.15 Structural formula of nicotinic acid (niacin).

"soft" CHD end-points; the cholestyramine-treatment group showed a 20% reduction in new-onset angina pectoris, a 25% decrease in positive exercise tests, and a 21% lowering of coronary artery surgery. When a life-table cumulative incidence of primary end-points was compared for placebo and cholestyramine groups, there was a two-year lag before a difference emerged, but thereafter the cumulative incidence diverged progressively in favor of the cholestyramine group (Fig. 4.13).

Further analysis of the results revealed that the reduction in coronary events was proportional to the decrease in LDL-cholesterol levels (Fig. 4.14). There was a wide range of responses, depending in part on drug compliance. Overall, it was estimated that a 1% decrease in cholesterol levels corresponded to an approximate 2% decrease in CHD risk. The results of this major clinical trial represent some of the strongest evidence that lowering serum total cholesterol (and LDL-cholesterol) reduces the risk for CHD.

NICOTINIC ACID

The B-vitamin nicotinic acid (niacin) has been used for many years as a cholesterol-lowering drug. Although nicotinic acid is a vitamin in low doses, it will not lower serum cholesterol levels at low intakes. Instead, it must be given in pharmacologic doses to produce a significant reduction in serum cholesterol concentrations. Therefore, when nicotinic acid is used as a cholesterol-lowering agent, it must be considered a drug and not a vitamin, and it should be administered only under the supervision of a physician.

AVAILABLE DRUGS

Nicotinic acid is the only currently available drug under this class of agent (Fig. 4.15). Several derivatives of nicotinic acid are presently under investigation, but none has been approved by the Food and Drug Administration in the United States for general use. Nicotinic acid is the least expensive of all lipid-lowering drugs, and it is available also as an "over-the-counter" drug, sold in health food stores as a vitamin. The quality of different brands of nicotinic acid may vary, particularly in their rates of bioavailability. Slow-release forms of nicotinic acid are available, and their use may reduce gastrointestinal side effects in some patients, although at the same time they may increase hepatotoxicity.

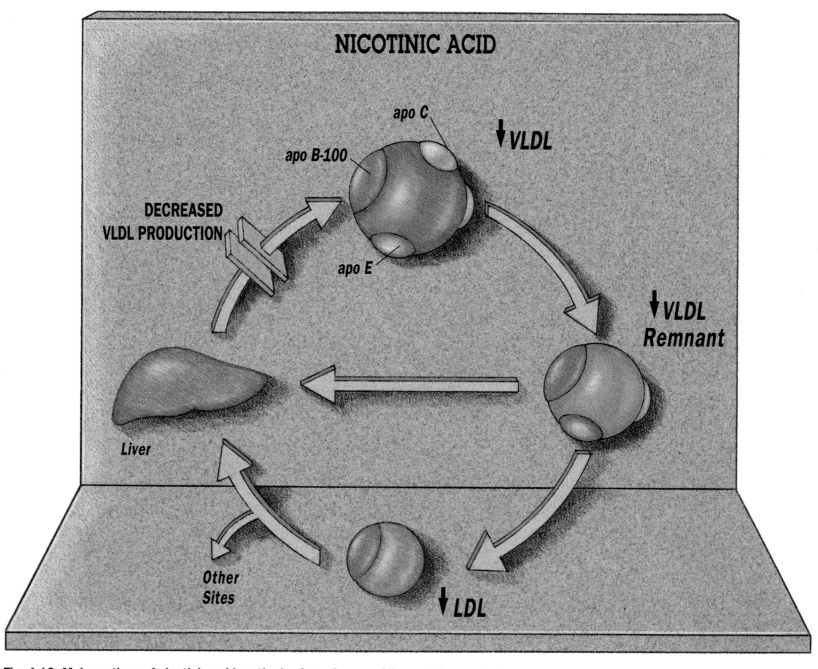

Fig. 4.16 Major actions of nicotinic acid on the basic pathways of lipoprotein metabolism.

MECHANISMS OF ACTION

The primary action of nicotinic acid is to inhibit the production of lipoproteins by the liver (Fig. 4.16). The mechanisms by which this occurs are unknown. The major consequence of this action is a decreased secretion of VLDL particles into the circulation, leading to a lowering of VLDL-triglyceride concentrations. Since VLDL particles are converted to LDL, nicotinic acid therapy al-so lowers levels of LDL-cholesterol in most patients. Reductions in serum LDL-cholesterol in the range of 15% to 25% are typical. The degree of LDL lowering generally is proportional to the dose, although there is considerable individual variability in response to the drug. Not only does nicotinic acid lower levels of lipoproteins containing apolipoprotein B (VLDL and LDL), but it also raises concentrations of HDL-cholesterol. The increase in the HDL fraction may be secondary to a decrease in VLDL-triglyceride concentrations (Fig. 4.17).

DOSAGE

The best responses to nicotinic acid therapy are obtained with intakes in the range of 3 to 6 g/day. An intake of 4.5 g (1500 mg three times daily), which is often used, usually is effective. Side effects are common with nicotinic

EFFECTS OF NICOTINIC ACID ON HDL-CHOLESTEROL

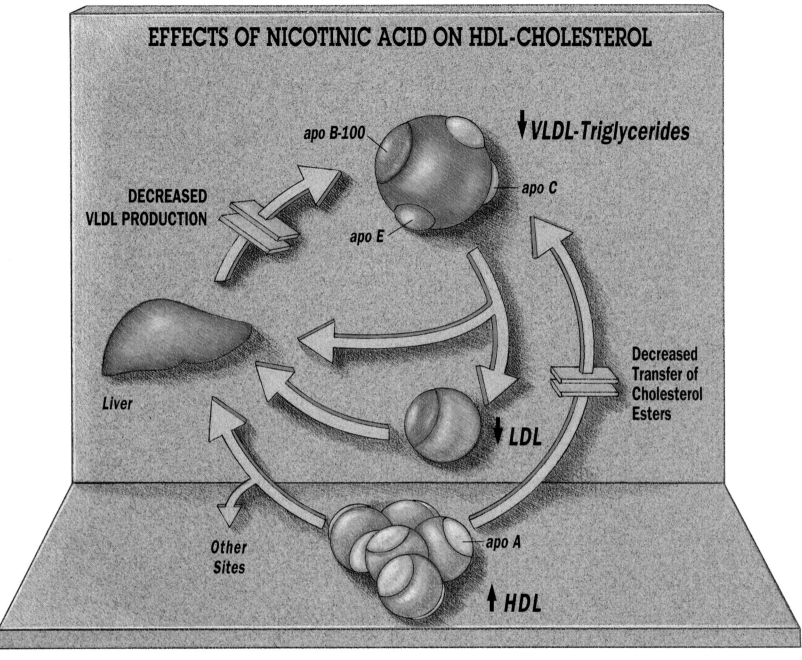

Fig. 4.17 Effects of reduced VLDL-triglyceride concentrations, secondary to nicotinic acid therapy, on HDL-cholesterol.

acid, but they may be minimized by starting the drug at low doses (e.g., 100 mg three times daily) and gradually increasing the dose over a period of weeks toward the therapeutic range.

SIDE EFFECTS

The major limitation to the use of nicotinic acid is the wide array of side effects it causes (Fig. 4.18). Only about 50% to 60% of patients are able to toler-

SIDE EFFECTS OF NICOTINIC ACID

GASTROINTESTINAL	SKIN	OTHER
Epigastric distress	Flushing	Hepatotoxicity
Activation of peptic ulcer	Itching	Glucose intolerance
Activation of chronic bowel disease	Skin rash	Hyperuricemia
	Acanthosis nigricans	Cardiac arrhythmias
		Toxic amblyopia

Fig. 4.18 Side effects of nicotinic acid.

Fig. 4.19 Indications for nicotinic acid.

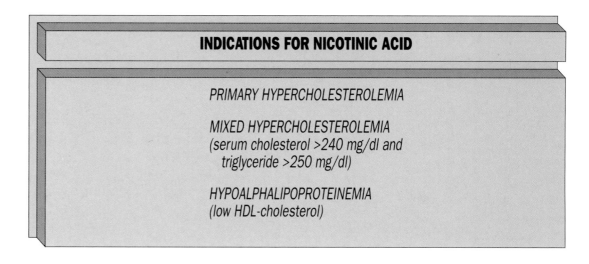

INDICATIONS FOR NICOTINIC ACID

PRIMARY HYPERCHOLESTEROLEMIA

MIXED HYPERCHOLESTEROLEMIA
(serum cholesterol >240 mg/dl and
triglyceride >250 mg/dl)

HYPOALPHALIPOPROTEINEMIA
(low HDL-cholesterol)

ate nicotinic acid on a long-term basis. To some extent, success with the drug depends on the motivations of both physicians and patients. The physician must understand the principles of administration of the drug, and the patient must recognize that there is potential benefit to be derived from nicotinic acid therapy and that side effects frequently disappear with prolonged usage.

Unfortunately, many patients taking nicotinic acid develop gastrointestinal side effects. Gastric irritation is the most common problem, and patients often complain of nausea and epigastric discomfort and/or burning. This effect often can be reduced by starting the drug in very low doses and increasing the dose very gradually. Nicotinic acid should not be taken on an empty stomach, but only with meals. Taking one dose with each meal, three times daily, may help to minimize gastric distress. Enteric-coated and timed-release forms of the drug likewise may mitigate gastrointestinal side effects. Nicotinic acid should not be given to patients with active peptic ulcer disease or inflammatory bowel disease. The drug must be used cautiously, if at all, in patients with a history of peptic ulcer disease.

Another side effect of nicotinic acid is flushing and itching of the skin. Flushing of the face is particularly common shortly after starting the drug, and typically it disappears over a period of time. Since this response is related to release of prostaglandins, it may be reduced by concomitant use of aspirin. Unacceptable itching is not unusual with nicotinic acid therapy, and skin rash occurs in a substantial number of patients. In rare instances, patients develop acanthosis nigricans during treatment with this drug.

Still another worrisome side effect is abnormality in liver function. Increases in transaminases are the most common manifestation. Apparently, nicotinic acid does not produce cirrhosis of the liver with prolonged therapy, but it may be prudent to withhold the drug in any patient who has significant and persistent elevation of liver enzymes. Recently, one case of massive hepatic necrosis due to high intakes of slow-release nicotinic acid was reported. Some patients develop a feeling of fatigue after prolonged ingestion of nicotinic acid. The reason for this response is not known, but most likely it is the result of subtle liver toxicity. When this occurs, it may be necessary to discontinue use of the drug. Nicotinic acid probably should not be used in combination therapy with inhibitors of HMG CoA reductase, because the latter are excreted through the liver; if liver changes induced by nicotinic acid interfere with excretion of reductase inhibitors, high blood levels of the latter can produce severe myopathy. (See discussion below on "HMG-CoA Reductase Inhibitors.")

Nicotinic acid induces metabolic side effects in some patients. It tends to worsen glucose tolerance, and in an occasional patient, it can precipitate frank diabetes mellitus. In diabetic patients, nicotinic acid can accentuate hyperglycemia; thus, for most diabetic patients, the drug probably should not be used even though it will improve the overall lipoprotein pattern. Nicotinic acid can increase uric acid levels and initiate an episode of acute gout in patients who already have a high serum uric acid.

It has been reported that nicotinic acid can cause arrhythmias in patients with established CHD; therefore, it should be used cautiously in such pa-

tients. Serious arrhythmias fortunately are relatively rare, but the physician must be aware of this possible adverse reaction in a patient with known CHD. Another rare side effect of nicotinic acid is toxic amblyopia.

INDICATIONS

Nicotinic acid is considered by many to be one of the drugs of first choice for treatment of hyperlipidemia, and it has several potential indications (Fig. 4.19). The drug is effective for lowering LDL-cholesterol levels in patients with primary hypercholesterolemia. Since it lowers triglycerides, it is useful for patients with mixed hyperlipidemia. Nicotinic acid, therefore, can be employed instead of a bile acid sequestrant if patients have mild hypertriglyceridemia in addition to elevated cholesterol concentrations. Although nicotinic acid raises HDL-cholesterol concentrations in hyperlipidemic patients, it remains to be shown that nicotinic acid effectively raises HDL-cholesterol levels in patients who have no other abnormalities in lipoprotein metabolism.

The efficacy of nicotinic acid for prevention of CHD was demonstrated in the Coronary Drug Project. All patients entering this trial already had established CHD. Those treated with nicotinic acid had fewer recurrent myocardial infarctions than patients treated with placebo. In the 15-year follow-up of patients in this study, those who had received nicotinic acid during the five years of the study had a lower all-causes mortality than did those in the placebo group. Thus, the efficacy of nicotinic acid in preventing CHD has been demonstrated, although its usefulness in practice is limited by a high incidence of side effects.

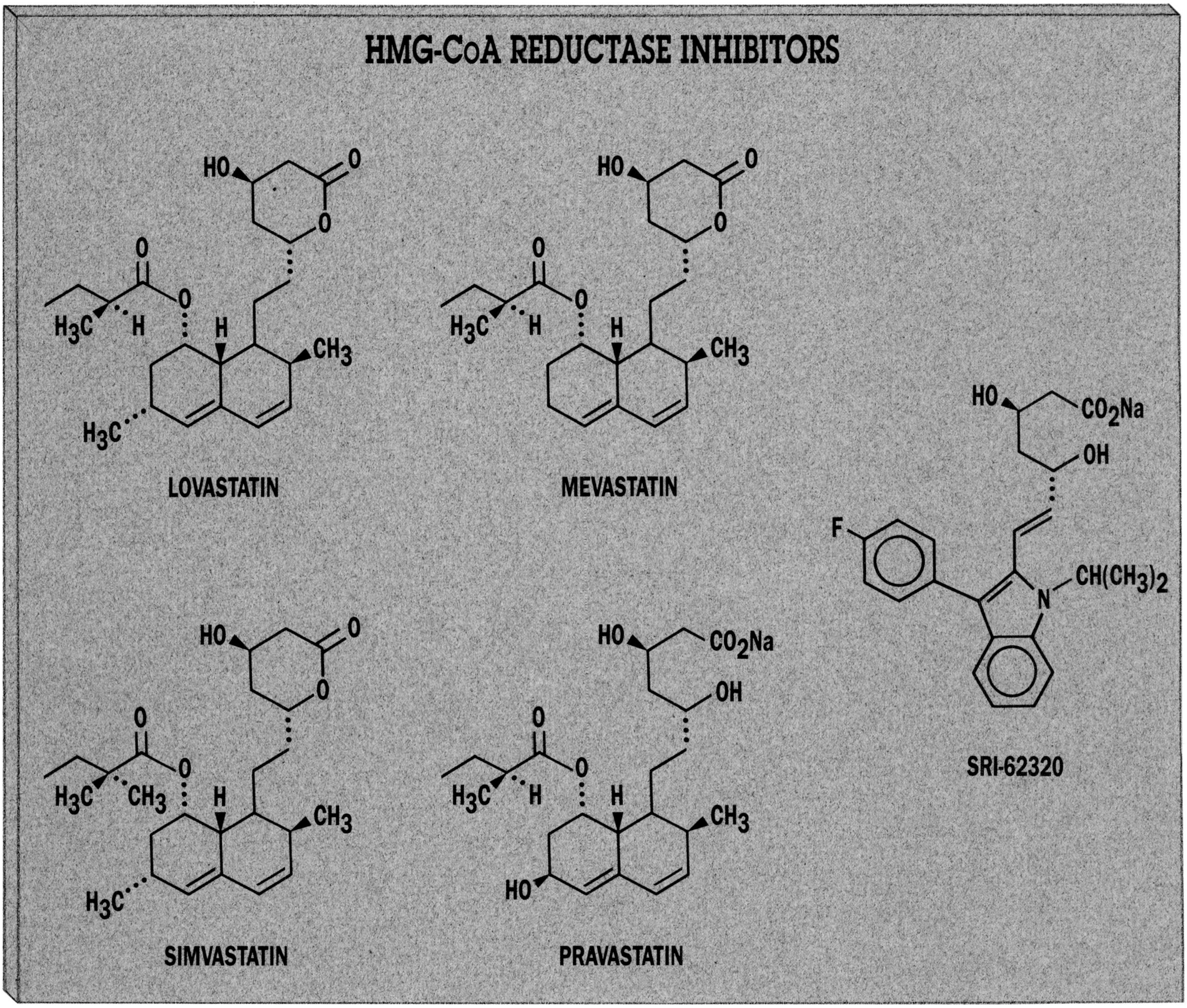

HMG-CoA REDUCTASE INHIBITORS

Fig. 4.20 Structural formulas of the HMG-CoA reductase inhibitors.

HMG-CoA REDUCTASE INHIBITORS

This new class of serum cholesterol-lowering drugs inhibits the rate-limiting enzyme in cholesterol synthesis, namely, 3-hydroxy-3-methylglutaryl coenzyme A (HMG CoA) reductase. These drugs are the most potent of all cholesterol-lowering agents, and thus far they have demonstrated few serious side effects. However, since they belong to a new class of drugs, their long-term safety has not been adequately proven;

and until their safety profile has been better defined, HMG-CoA reductase inhibitors must be used with caution. They are best reserved for patients with severe elevations of LDL-cholesterol or those with moderate hypercholesterolemia who are at high risk for CHD from other causes.

AVAILABLE DRUGS

Several HMG-CoA reductase inhibitors are currently being used or developed (Fig. 4.20). The first drug of this class

was mevastatin. It was discovered in Japan in 1976, and shortly thereafter it was shown to reduce serum cholesterol levels in both experimental animals and man. The first agent to become available in the United States was lovastatin, which was approved by the Food and Drug Administration for treatment of hypercholesterolemia in 1987. Other HMG-CoA reductase inhibitors, notably pravastatin and simvastatin, are in clinical studies and will be available in the next few years.

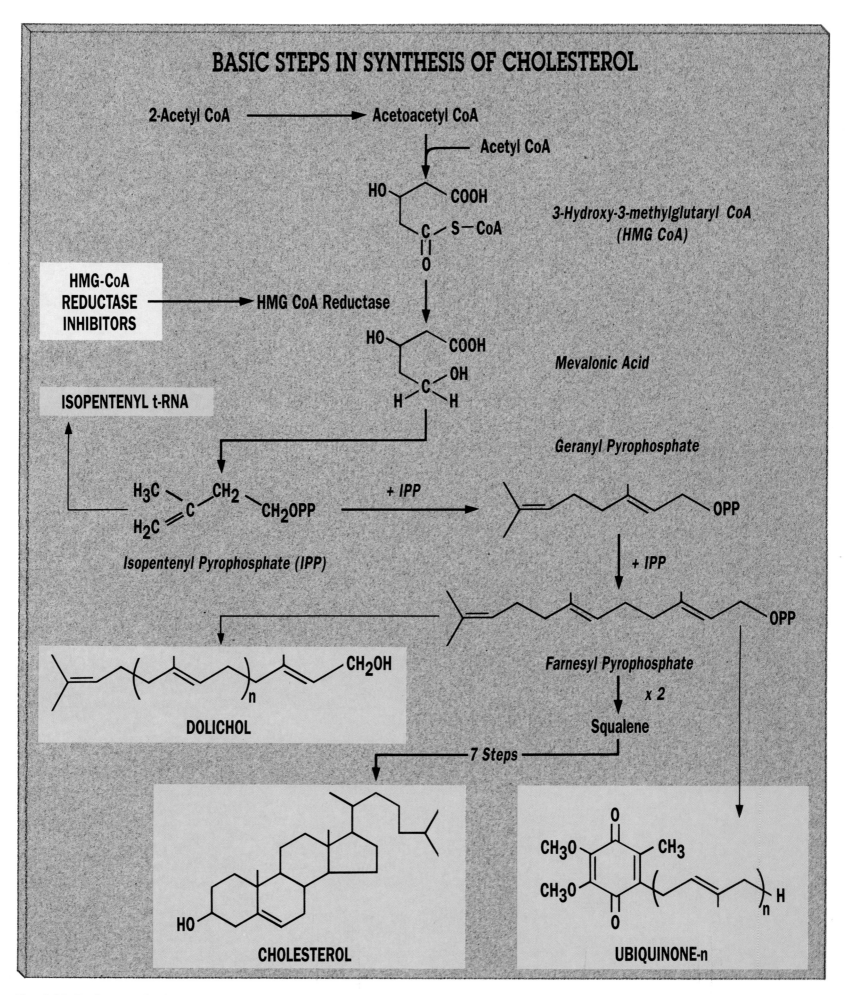

BASIC STEPS IN SYNTHESIS OF CHOLESTEROL

Fig. 4.21 Basic steps in the synthesis of cholesterol, showing the site of action of HMG-CoA reductase inhibitors.

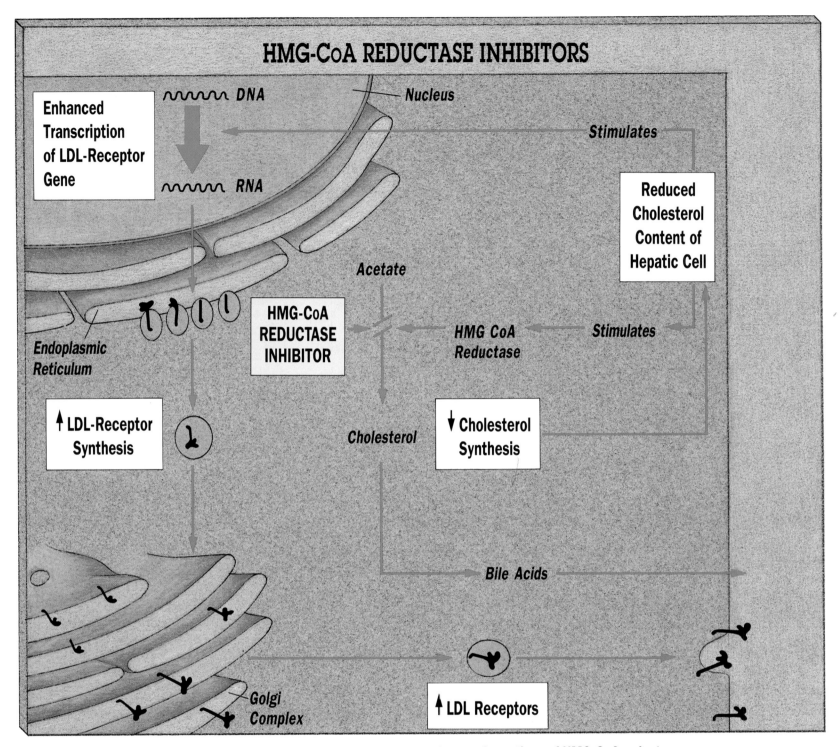

HMG-CoA REDUCTASE INHIBITORS

Enhanced Transcription of LDL-Receptor Gene

DNA

Nucleus

RNA

Stimulates

Reduced Cholesterol Content of Hepatic Cell

Acetate

Endoplasmic Reticulum

HMG-CoA REDUCTASE INHIBITOR

HMG CoA Reductase

Stimulates

↑ LDL-Receptor Synthesis

Cholesterol

↓ Cholesterol Synthesis

Bile Acids

Golgi Complex

↑ LDL Receptors

Fig. 4.22 Effects of reduced cholesterol content of hepatic cells, secondary to the actions of HMG-CoA reductase inhibitors, on the synthesis of cholesterol and LDL receptors.

MECHANISMS OF ACTION

The basic steps in the synthesis of cholesterol and other products of mevalonic acid, as well as the site of action of HMG-CoA reductase inhibitors, are presented in Figure 4.21. Theoretically, inhibition of HMG CoA reductase should reduce formation of all products of mevalonic acid, namely, cholesterol, dolichol, ubiquinone, and isopentenyl adenine. Investigations have shown that the synthesis of cholesterol is partially inhibited in humans by these drugs, but the degree of cholesterol-synthesis inhibition is inadequate to produce a deficiency of whole-body cholesterol. No data indicate that these drugs significantly reduce other products of mevalonic acid in humans.

The primary action of HMG-CoA reductase inhibitors is to lower the level of serum LDL-cholesterol. This action is mediated mainly through stimulation of LDL-receptor activity. By inhibiting the synthesis of cholesterol in the liver, these drugs reverse the inhibitory effect of elevated hepatic cholesterol on LDL-receptor synthesis; as a result, the number of cell-surface receptors increases markedly (Fig. 4.22). The increase in LDL-receptor activity occurs mainly in the liver. This causes a fall in LDL levels in two ways: by promoting the direct uptake of circulating LDL by the liver and by enhancing hepatic uptake of

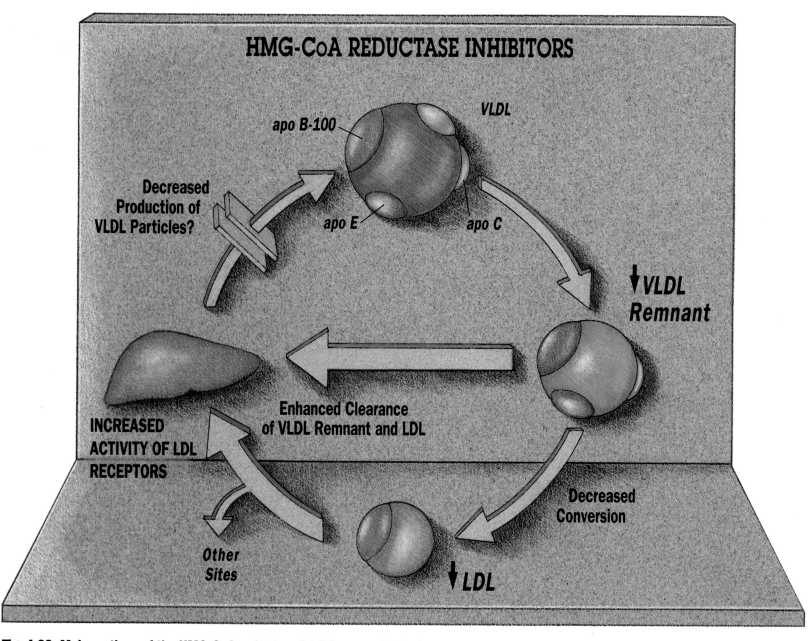

Fig. 4.23 Major actions of the HMG-CoA reductase inhibitors on the basic pathways of lipoprotein metabolism.

Fig. 4.24 Side effects of HMG-CoA reductase inhibitors.

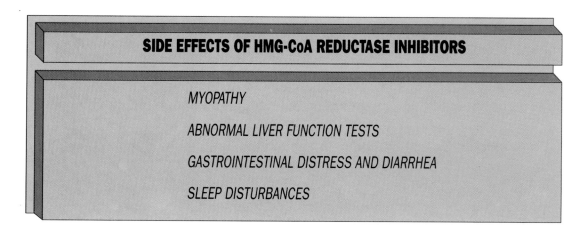

MYOPATHY INDUCED BY HMG-CoA REDUCTASE INHIBITORS

INTERMITTENT MUSCLE WEAKNESS AND TENDERNESS

ELEVATIONS OF SERUM CREATINE KINASE

SEVERE MYOPATHY (rare)
  SIGNS:
  Marked proximal muscle weakness and tenderness
  Extreme elevations of creatine kinase
  Myoglobinuria
  Acute renal failure

  PRECIPITATING FACTORS:
  Liver disease
  Concomitant drug use (cyclosporine, gemfibrozil, nicotinic acid)

Fig. 4.25 Clinical features of myopathy induced by HMG-CoA reductase inhibitors.

VLDL and VLDL remnants, the precursors of LDL (Fig. 4.23). Because of the latter, fewer VLDL are converted to LDL, thereby assisting in the decrease in LDL levels.

Some investigators have speculated that HMG-CoA reductase inhibitors also decrease hepatic synthesis of lipoproteins, possibly because they reduce availability of cholesterol for formation of lipoproteins. Support for this concept comes from the observation that reductase inhibitors lower concentrations of VLDL in many patients. If this mechanism pertains, part of the fall in LDL levels could be the result of decreased formation of VLDL, the precursor of LDL. On the other hand, a decrease in serum VLDL-triglycerides, commonly noted with reductase-inhibitor therapy, could be the result of enhanced direct removal of VLDL and VLDL remnants. The triglyceride-lowering action of HMG-CoA reductase inhibitors is relatively modest compared with their effects on LDL-cholesterol.

Finally, HMG-CoA reductase inhibitors will raise HDL-cholesterol levels in some patients. Just how this occurs is not known, although this response also has been reported for bile acid sequestrants, which likewise increase the activity of LDL receptors. The degree of rise in HDL levels by reductase inhibitors generally is modest.

DOSAGE

The different reductase inhibitors vary in their ability to inhibit HMG CoA reductase, and consequently their dosage can vary. Lovastatin generally is given as 20 mg/day or 20 mg twice daily. Reductions of LDL-cholesterol in the range of 25% to 30% usually occur with the lower dose, whereas decreases of 30% to 35% are found at the higher dose. An even higher dose—40 mg twice daily—can lower LDL-cholesterol up to 40%, although this high dose is not required for most patients; moreover, it is costly and may be associated with more side effects.

SIDE EFFECTS

To date the HMG-CoA reductase inhibitors have been relatively free of serious side effects (Fig. 4.24). As indicated before, however, they have not been tested in individual patients for many years, and long-term side effects may yet emerge.

The most common side effect of reductase inhibitors is myopathy, which can occur in three forms (Fig. 4.25). First, about 5% of patients will complain of intermittent muscle weakness and tenderness. This usually is transitory, and is not always accompanied by elevations of serum creatine kinase. In

Fig. 4.26 Indications for HMG-CoA reductase inhibitors.

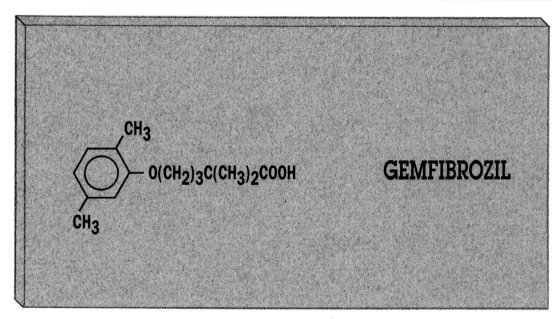

INDICATIONS FOR HMG-CoA REDUCTASE INHIBITORS

SEVERE HYPERCHOLESTEROLEMIA
Heterozygous FH
Severe nonfamilial hypercholesterolemia

MODERATE HYPERCHOLESTEROLEMIA IN HIGH-RISK PATIENTS
Established CHD
Persistent smoking
Diabetes mellitus
Low HDL-cholesterol

Fig. 4.27 Structural formula of gemfibrozil.

$O(CH_2)_3C(CH_3)_2COOH$

GEMFIBROZIL

some cases, it is difficult to be certain that muscle symptoms are due to the drug, but these symptoms appear to be more common in patients taking reductase inhibitors than in untreated subjects. Second, another 5% of patients will have intermittent increases in creatine kinase, with or without muscle symptoms. Increases in creatine kinase often are transitory, and for most patients, they may not require discontinuance of the drug. And third, about 0.2% of patients will develop more severe myopathy. Occasionally, patients may manifest severe muscle weakness, extreme elevations of creatine kinase, myoglobinuria, and even acute tubular necrosis. This severe reaction rarely may occur in patients taking only reductase inhibitors without concomitant inhibiting factors, but it is more

likely to occur in the presence of other drugs or diseases; specifically, severe myopathy may occur with simultaneous use of cyclosporine, fibric acids (e.g., gemfibrozil), and nicotinic acid, or in the presence of liver disease.

A second side effect is a rise in liver enzymes, usually transaminases. Whether this response represents hepatic toxicity is unknown. The increases in hepatic enzymes almost always return to normal on removal of the drug. It is not known whether prolonged administration of HMG-CoA reductase inhibitors in the face of elevated hepatic enzymes will produce chronic liver disease.

HMG-CoA reductase inhibitors can cause various gastrointestinal symptoms, most commonly diarrhea. They also have been reported to cause insomnia or other sleep disturbances in

occasional patients. Of greater concern is the development of cataracts, which does occur at very high doses in dogs. Careful studies in humans, however, have yielded no evidence of cataract formation at the usual therapeutic doses.

INDICATIONS

The HMG-CoA reductase inhibitors have several potential indications (Fig. 4.26). They are especially valuable for severe elevations of LDL-cholesterol, as in heterozygous FH and other forms of primary severe hypercholesterolemia. Because of the high risk for CHD associated with these conditions, the use of reductase inhibitors can be justified even though insufficient information is available on long-term side effects. It

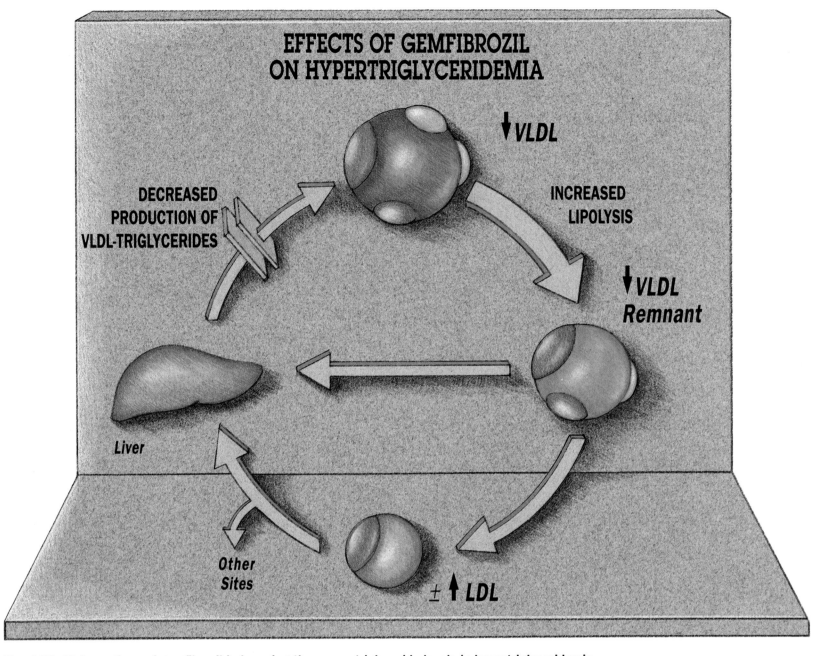

**EFFECTS OF GEMFIBROZIL
ON HYPERTRIGLYCERIDEMIA**

↓VLDL

INCREASED
LIPOLYSIS

DECREASED
PRODUCTION OF
VLDL-TRIGLYCERIDES

↓VLDL
Remnant

Liver

Other
Sites

± ↑ LDL

Fig. 4.28 Major actions of gemfibrozil in lowering the serum triglyceride levels in hypertriglyceridemia.

also is reasonable to consider therapy with HMG-CoA reductase inhibitors in patients with moderately elevated concentrations of LDL-cholesterol who are at high risk for CHD from other factors, e.g., persistent smoking, established CHD, reduced HDL-cholesterol, familial combined hyperlipidemia (see Figs. 2.33, 2.34), or dysbetalipoproteinemia (type III HLP; see Fig. 2.19). They also may be efficacious in patients with diabetic dyslipidemia (see Fig. 2.40) or the nephrotic syndrome (see Figs. 2.37, 2.38). It may be premature, however,

to consider use of these drugs in patients with moderate elevations of LDL-cholesterol in the absence of other risk factors.

GEMFIBROZIL

Gemfibrozil is a lipid-lowering drug that is structurally similar to the fibric acids (Fig. 4.27). It dramatically lowers serum triglycerides in patients with hypertriglyceridemia, but it also can reduce LDL-cholesterol levels in patients without hypertriglyceridemia. Gemfibrozil

also causes a rise in serum HDL-cholesterol levels in most patients.

MECHANISMS OF ACTION

The action of gemfibrozil in lowering serum triglycerides has been attributed to two actions (Fig. 4.28). First, it interferes with the synthesis of VLDL-triglycerides in the liver; and second, it appears to increase the activity of lipoprotein lipase. Whether both of these actions are primary and independent of one another has not been determined.

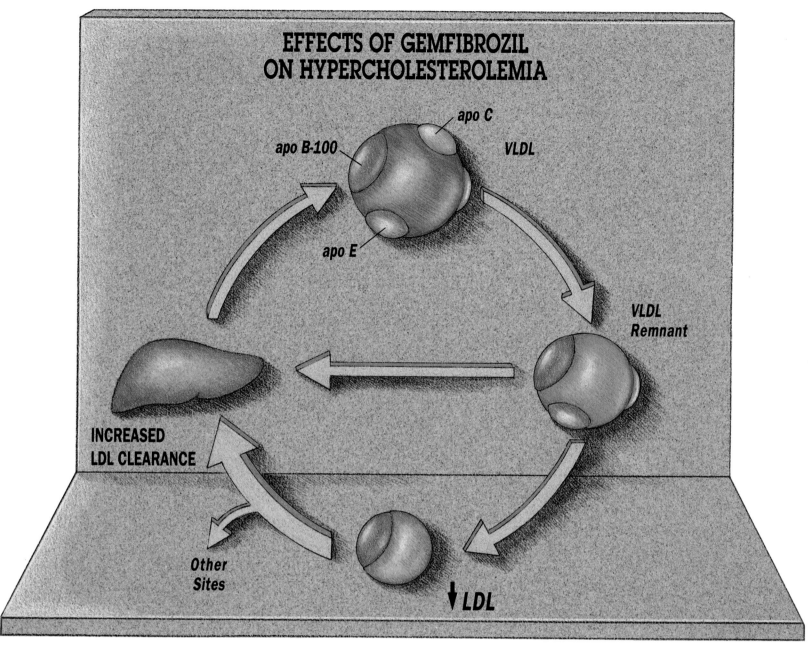

EFFECTS OF GEMFIBROZIL ON HYPERCHOLESTEROLEMIA

apo C

apo B-100

VLDL

apo E

VLDL Remnant

INCREASED LDL CLEARANCE

Other Sites

↓ LDL

Fig. 4.29 Major actions of gemfibrozil in lowering the LDL-cholesterol levels in hypercholesterolemia.

Regardless, the drug seemingly promotes the lipolysis of both VLDL-triglycerides and chylomicron triglycerides and can dramatically lower triglyceride levels.

Another action of gemfibrozil is to lower LDL-cholesterol concentrations. Limited data suggest that the drug causes a mild increase in activity of LDL receptors, thereby promoting the clearance of circulating LDL (Fig. 4.29).

In patients with primary hypercholesterolemia, decreases in LDL-cholesterol in the range of 10% to 15% are typical. In patients with hypertriglyceridemia, on the other hand, gemfibrozil sometimes raises LDL-cholesterol concentrations simultaneously with a lowering of serum triglycerides. In these patients, total cholesterol levels often are not altered; instead, cholesterol in VLDL is shifted to LDL.

In contrast, in patients with mixed hyperlipidemia (elevated triglyceride and cholesterol levels), decreases in VLDL-triglycerides frequently are accompanied by a reduction in serum LDL-cholesterol. Thus, in mixed hyperlipidemia, high levels of LDL-cholesterol often are reduced, whether or not they are accompanied by increased serum concentrations of VLDL-triglycerides.

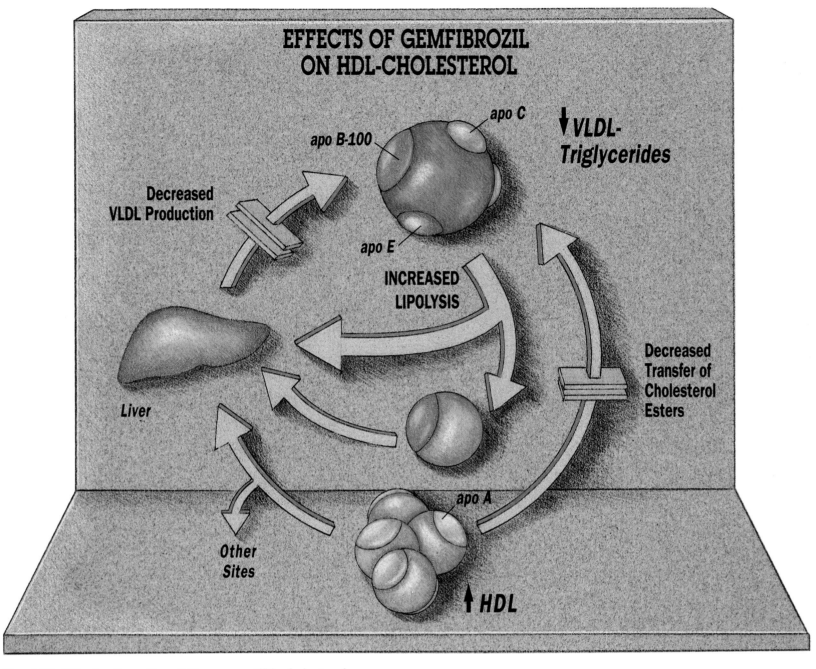

EFFECTS OF GEMFIBROZIL ON HDL-CHOLESTEROL

apo C

apo B-100

↓VLDL-Triglycerides

Decreased VLDL Production

apo E

INCREASED LIPOLYSIS

Decreased Transfer of Cholesterol Esters

Liver

apo A

Other Sites

↑ HDL

Fig. 4.30 Effects of gemfibrozil therapy on HDL-cholesterol.

Finally, gemfibrozil usually causes an increase in HDL-cholesterol concentrations. The rise in serum HDL-cholesterol typically ranges between 10% and 25%. The mechanism for this rise is unknown, but it may be secondary to decreased VLDL-triglyceride production and enhanced activity of lipoprotein lipase (Fig. 4.30). Because of the inverse relation between VLDL-triglyceride and HDL-cholesterol concentrations, a fall in the former will result in a rise in the latter.

DOSAGE

The recommended dosage of gemfibrozil is 1200 mg daily. It usually is given in divided doses of 600 mg each, administered 30 minutes before morning and evening meals. It may be appropriate to reduce the dose in patients with renal disease, as required for other fibric acids, but limited experience is available on this point.

SIDE EFFECTS

Gemfibrozil therapy is accompanied by an increased risk for cholesterol gall-

Fig. 4.31 Side effects of gemfibrozil.

SIDE EFFECTS OF GEMFIBROZIL

CHOLESTEROL GALLSTONES

MYOPATHY

EPIGASTRIC DISTRESS

OTHER
Potentiation of anticoagulant
    action of warfarin
Leukopenia
Increased hepatic enzymes

Fig. 4.32 Possible indications for gemfi-brozil.

POSSIBLE INDICATIONS FOR GEMFIBROZIL

TYPE V HLP
(increased VLDL and chylomicrons)

TYPE III HLP (DYSBETALIPOPROTEINEMIA)
(increased beta-VLDL)

TYPE IIB HLP
(increased VLDL and LDL)

TYPE IIA HLP
(increased LDL)

TYPE IV
(increased VLDL)

HYPOALPHALIPOPROTEINEMIA
(decreased HDL)

stones (Fig. 4.31). It can cause supersaturation of bile with cholesterol, a change resulting from partial inhibition of synthesis of bile acids and increased secretion of cholesterol into bile. Approximately 2% to 4% of patients treated with gemfibrozil may develop gallstones.

A second side effect of gemfibrozil therapy is myopathy. Patients may complain of muscle weakness and tenderness, together with elevations of creatine kinase. The degree of myopathy generally is mild when the patient is taking only gemfibrozil, and it subsides rapidly once the drug is discontinued. The danger of myopathy may be increased in patients with chronic renal failure. The combination of gemfibrozil with a HMG-CoA reductase inhibitor is associated with an increased risk for severe myopathy (see Fig. 4.25), which can occur in approximately one in 20 patients. Therefore, either this combination should be avoided, or patients receiving the combination must be monitored carefully.

Another adverse reaction is gastrointestinal distress, most often gastric irritation. A variety of other side effects has been reported; these include potentiation of anticoagulant action of warfarin; leukopenia; impotence; weight gain; and increases in hepatic enzymes. In general, gemfibrozil should be withheld in pregnant women or nursing mothers, unless it is required for prevention of acute pancreatitis due to severe hypertriglyceridemia.

INDICATIONS

Gemfibrozil has several potential indications (Fig. 4.32). One clear indication for gemfibrozil therapy is prevention of acute pancreatitis in patients with severe hypertriglyceridemia. The most common reason for triglyceride levels over 1000 mg/dl is type V hyperlipoproteinemia (HLP), in which both VLDL and chylomicrons are increased (see Fig. 2.21). Gemfibrozil treatment can be considered when dietary therapy alone does not successfully lower serum triglyceride levels to below 1000 mg/dl, or preferably, to below 500 mg/dl. Patients with type V HLP presumably have reduced but not absent lipoprotein-lipase activity that can be enhanced by gemfibrozil therapy. Some patients with type V HLP are resistant to gemfibrozil treatment, possibly because of markedly reduced lipoprotein-lipase activity, which does

not respond to the action of the drug. It should be noted that type IV HLP in some patients can be rapidly converted to type V HLP, thereby putting them at risk for pancreatitis, and, therefore, type IV patients with triglyceride levels in the range of 500 to 1000 mg/dl are candidates for gemfibrozil therapy. On the other hand, in patients with type I HLP (see Fig. 2.17), who have a complete absence of lipoprotein lipase, gemfibrozil is ineffective in mitigating the chylomicronemia.

Another reason to use gemfibrozil therapy is to reduce the risk for CHD in patients with various forms of dyslipidemia. In general, consideration should be given first to use of a bile acid sequestrant or nicotinic acid. If these drugs, or perhaps a HMG-CoA reductase inhibitor, are not well tolerated or efficacious for serum lipid lowering, gemfibrozil can be considered. The rationale for use of gemfibrozil therapy for prevention of CHD comes mainly from the Helsinki Heart Study. This study, a large, randomized, double-blind, placebo-controlled primary prevention trial, was carried out in 4,081 Finnish men between the ages of 40 and 55. The participants in this trial had elevated total cholesterol levels oc-

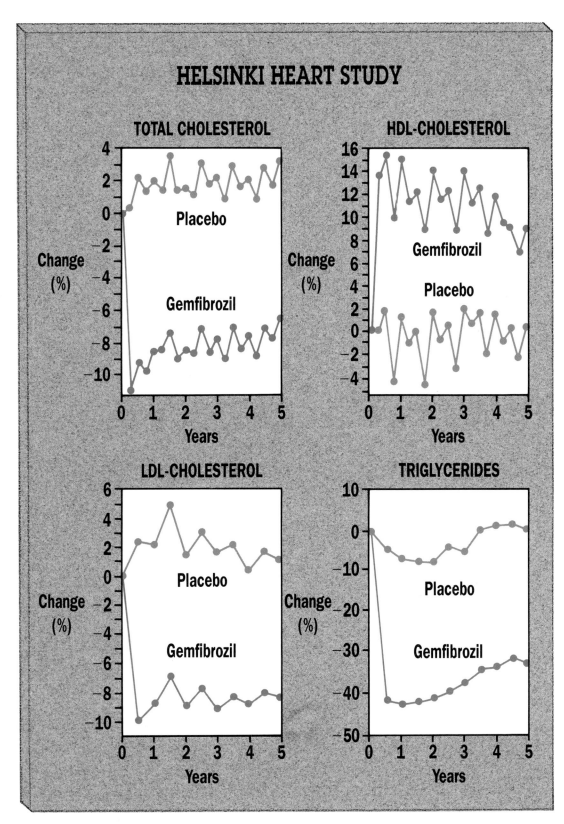

Fig. 4.33 Comparison of changes in lipid values from baseline in the placebo and gemfibrozil groups participating in the Helsinki Heart Study.

curring in several patterns, i.e., types IIA, IIB, and IV HLP (see Figs. 2.15, 2.16). For all participants in this study, the non-HDL-cholesterol level was over 200 mg/dl at baseline, and none of the patients had a history of previous CHD. For the group as a whole, therapy caused a moderate lowering of serum total cholesterol and LDL-cholesterol, a reduction in serum triglycerides, and a rise in HDL-cholesterol levels (Fig. 4.33).

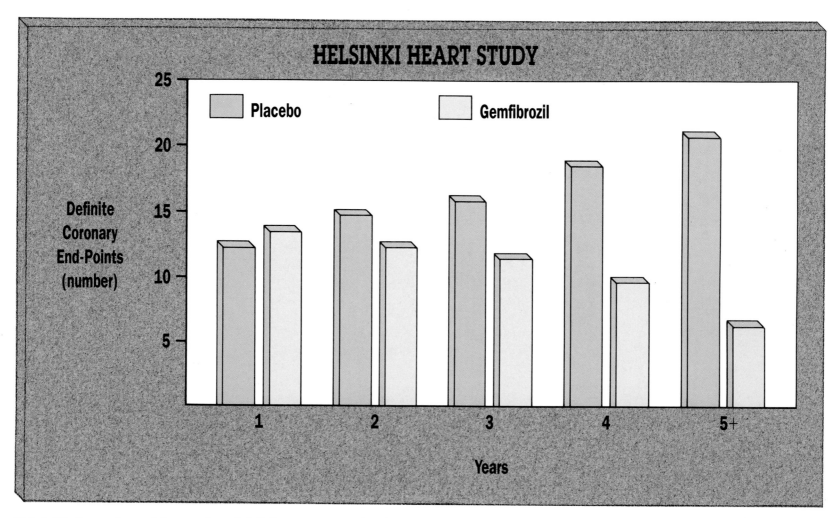

Fig. 4.34 Comparison of the number of definite coronary end-points in the placebo and gemfibrozil groups in the Helsinki Heart Study.

Over the five-year period of this trial, the gemfibrozil-therapy group had a 34% reduction in serious coronary events (sudden coronary deaths plus fatal and nonfatal myocardial infarctions) compared with placebo. There was a two-year lag before benefit became manifest, but thereafter the gemfibrozil-treated group showed a progressive decline in CHD rates compared with placebo (Fig. 4.34). Nonfatal myocardial infarctions for the entire study were reduced by 37%. No ev-

idence was obtained of increased non-cardiovascular mortality in the gemfibrozil group, nor were serious, life-threatening side effects observed.

On the basis of the Helsinki Heart Study, one indication for gemfibrozil therapy for the purpose of reducing CHD risk is for patients with type IIB HLP. About one fourth of the patients entering the Helsinki Heart Study had this phenotype. The greatest reduction in incidence of serious coronary events occurred in type IIB HLP patients, who

had elevations of both LDL-cholesterol and total serum triglycerides. These patients had lower HDL-cholesterol levels than type IIA HLP patients, and the percentage increase in HDL-cholesterol levels in patients with type IIB HLP was 12.6%.

Another potential indication for gemfibrozil therapy is type IIA HLP. Patients of this type constituted the largest subgroup of hypercholesterolemic individuals in the Helsinki Heart Study. The type IIA patients likewise had a reduc-

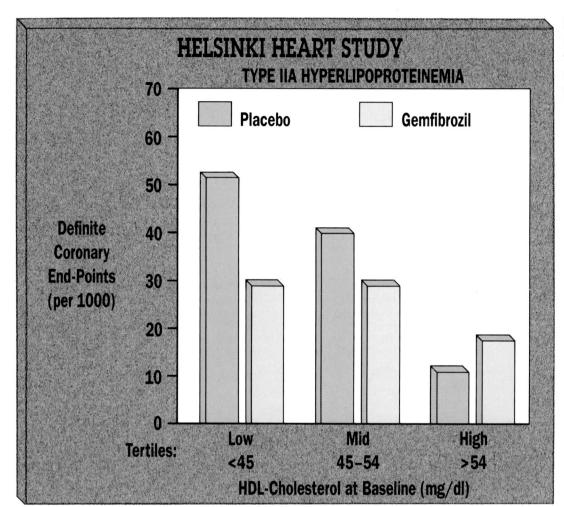

HELSINKI HEART STUDY
TYPE IIA HYPERLIPOPROTEINEMIA

Placebo **Gemfibrozil**

Definite Coronary End-Points (per 1000)

Tertiles:
Low <45
Mid 45–54
High >54

HDL-Cholesterol at Baseline (mg/dl)

Fig. 4.35 Comparison of the incidence of definite coronary end-points by HDL-cholesterol tertiles at baseline in placebo- and gemfibrozil-treated individuals identified as having type IIA HLP in the Helsinki Heart Study.

tion in CHD rates with gemfibrozil therapy, compared with the placebo group. In patients with type IIA HLP, reductions in LDL-cholesterol levels of 10% to 15% are typical with gemfibrozil therapy. The response to gemfibrozil therapy often is greater in patients with higher LDL-cholesterol concentrations.

Among the type IIA patients in the Helsinki Heart Study, reduction in coronary end-points depended on baseline levels of both LDL and HDL. Thus, the mean decrease in coronary end-points in patients receiving gemfibrozil occurred in those with HDL-cholesterol levels in the lowest tertile at baseline (Fig. 4.35). This finding adds justifiction

for use of gemfibrozil in patients with combined lipoprotein defects, i.e., high LDL and low HDL levels. This pattern, of course, is associated with high ratios of total cholesterol to HDL-cholesterol, or LDL-cholesterol to HDL-cholesterol.

Another potential indication for gemfibrozil therapy is type IV HLP. In the Helsinki Heart Study, gemfibrozil treatment of subjects with this phenotype appeared to reduce cardiac end-points. It must be noted, however, that in spite of this trend, the number of participants with type IV HLP in the Helsinki Heart Study was inadequate to achieve statistical significance. In type IV HLP, gemfibrozil is highly effective for lower-

ing VLDL-triglyceride concentrations, but it generally does not lower serum apolipoprotein-B levels and may increase LDL-cholesterol concentrations. Gemfibrozil therapy usually raises HDL-cholesterol levels by 10% to 25% in patients with type IV HLP.

Gemfibrozil therapy usually is highly effective for treatment of familial dysbetalipoproteinemia (type III HLP) (see Fig. 2.19). Patients with this condition have elevations in both triglycerides and cholesterol in the VLDL fraction (beta-VLDL), and both lipids are lowered by treatment with gemfibrozil. In many type III patients, lipid levels are completely normalized.

Fig. 4.36 Comparison of changes from base-line in the LDL-C/HDL-C ratios for placebo and gemfibrozil groups in the Helsinki Heart Study.

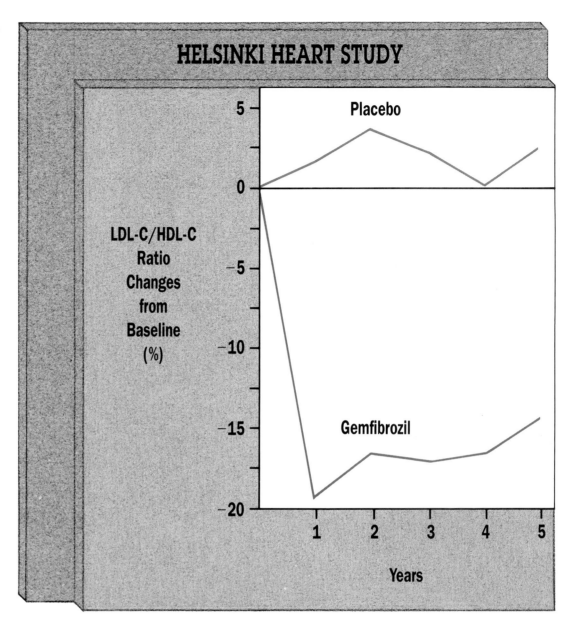

Finally, consideration should be given to use of gemfibrozil for treatment of low serum HDL-cholesterol, especially when low levels of HDL are combined with an increase in LDL-cholesterol concentrations. With this combined abnormality, gemfibrozil produces an improvement in the LDL-C/HDL-C ratio, as was noted in the Helsinki Heart Study (Fig. 4.36). Whether gemfibrozil is indicated for patients with an isolated decrease in HDL-cholesterol in the presence of normal serum total cholesterol and triglycerides is not known. It might be noted, however, that the rise in HDL-cholesterol levels in patients receiving gemfibrozil in the Helsinki Heart Study was estimated to be one reason for the decrease in CHD risk in this group.

OTHER FIBRIC ACIDS

Other drugs in the class of fibric acids have been used for many years throughout the world for treatment of dyslipidemia. These drugs include clofibrate, fenofibrate, bezafibrate, and ciprofibrate (Fig. 4.37). Clofibrate, the first available fibric acid, has been used extensively for about 25 years. It has been approved by the Food and Drug Administration in the United States for the purpose of lowering severely elevated triglyceride levels, but not for routine therapy of elevated serum cholesterol concentrations to reduce the risk for CHD. The efficacy and safety of clofibrate have been tested in two major clinical trials. In the Coronary Drug Project, which was a secondary prevention trial, clofibrate therapy caused a modest lowering in serum total cholesterol levels, but did not alter the recurrence rate for myocardial infarction in comparison with rates in the placebo-treated group. Clofibrate also was tested in hypercholesterolemic subjects in the World Health Organization study, which was a primary prevention trial. Although clofibrate decreased the rate of myocardial infarction, compared with placebo, it did not improve overall mortality. In fact, mortality was slightly higher in the drug-treatment group than in the placebo group, suggesting that the drug carries an inherent toxicity. Because of the unfavorable results of the World Health Organization trial, use of clofibrate for treatment of hyperlipidemia has declined steadily in the past few years.

The other fibric acids shown in Figure 4.37 are available for use in many countries but not in the United States. Fenofibrate differs from clofibrate by replacement of the chloride atom with a parachlorobenzoyl group. The drug was first made available in France about 15 years ago, and is now widely used in other countries. It is more potent than clofibrate and requires smaller doses for the same lipid-lowering effect. Bezafibrate has a similar potency as fenofibrate, and it differs from clofibrate by inclusion of a benzamidoethyl group. The actions of these fibric acids on lipid and lipoprotein metabolism are similar to those outlined for gemfibrozil (see Figs. 4.28–4.30). The claim has been made that fenofibrate and bezafibrate are more effective in lower-

OTHER FIBRIC ACIDS

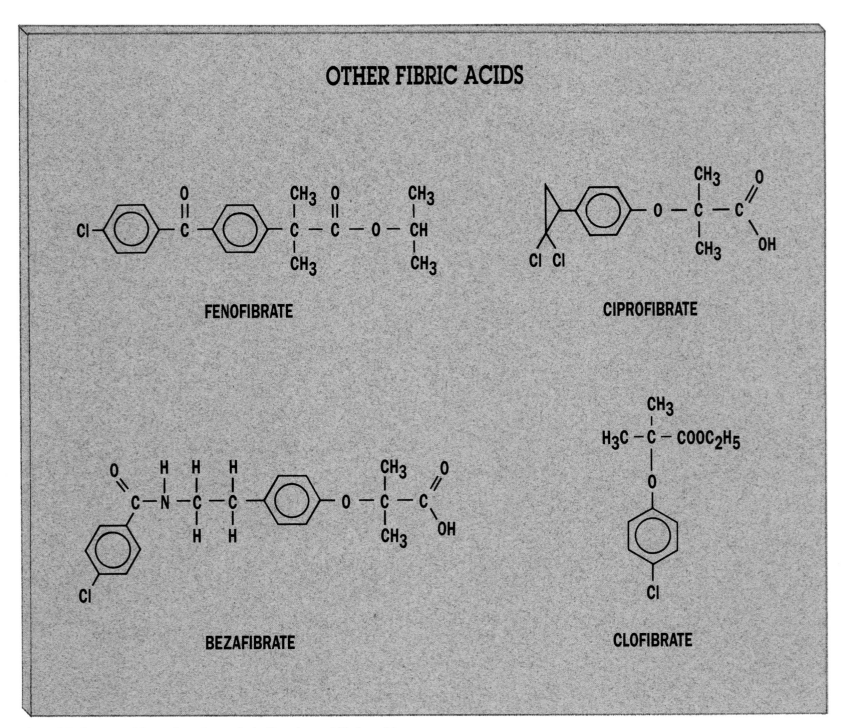

FENOFIBRATE

CIPROFIBRATE

BEZAFIBRATE

CLOFIBRATE

Fig. 4.37 Structural formulas of agents in the class of fibric acids.

ing LDL-cholesterol levels than clofibrate and gemfibrozil, but this claim has not been confirmed by direct comparison studies. The side-effect profile of all fibric acids appears similar.

PROBUCOL

Probucol is a cholesterol-lowering drug that has been approved by the Food and Drug Administration for LDL-cholesterol lowering (Fig. 4.38). It causes only a modest reduction in LDL levels, and it has not been tested for safety and efficacy in a large clinical trial. Recent studies indicate that probucol prevents the oxidation of LDL, and through this mechanism, it may slow development of coronary atherosclerosis.

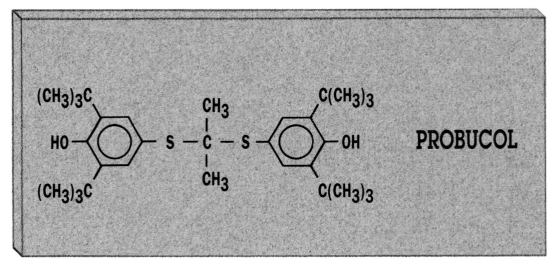

PROBUCOL

Fig. 4.38 Structural formula of probucol.

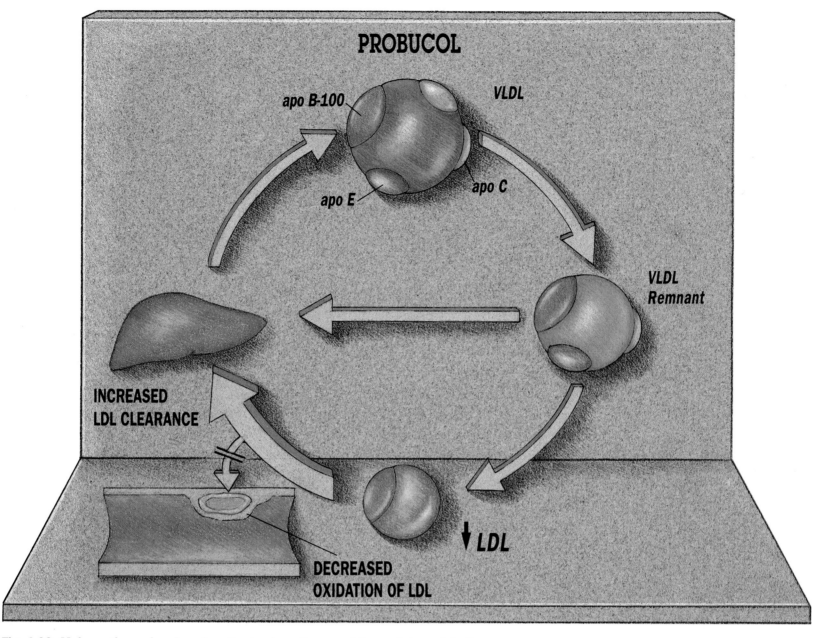

PROBUCOL

apo B-100

VLDL

apo E

apo C

VLDL
Remnant

INCREASED
LDL CLEARANCE

↓ LDL

DECREASED
OXIDATION OF LDL

Fig. 4.39 Major actions of probucol on the basic pathways of lipoprotein metabolism.

MECHANISMS OF ACTION

The precise mechanism whereby probucol acts to lower levels of LDL-cholesterol is not known. However, studies of LDL metabolism in humans indicate that probucol promotes the clearance of LDL from the circulation (Fig. 4.39). Whether enhanced clearance of LDL occurs via LDL-receptor or nonreceptor pathways is not known. Since probucol appears to reduce LDL levels in patients with homozygous FH, who have no LDL receptors, increased clearance of LDL may occur via nonreceptor pathways; this, however, has not been demonstrated. Probucol lowers the LDL-cholesterol concentrations by approximately 15%.

Another action of probucol is to reduce HDL-cholesterol levels by 15% to 25%. Several studies suggest that the HDL-lowering action is related to decreased synthesis of apolipoprotein A-I. There is a general concern that the reduction in HDL levels may offset the benefit to be derived from lowering the LDL-cholesterol concentration with probucol therapy.

Probucol is a lipid-soluble drug, and it apparently is carried within lipoprotein particles. The drug also is an antioxidant and, therefore, prevents the oxidation of LDL. One theory of atherosclerosis holds that oxidation of LDL is a key first step in the development of foam cells, the hallmark of atherosclerotic lesions. Oxidized LDL are more readily

taken up by macrophages than native LDL, and prevention of LDL oxidation by probucol may retard development of atherosclerosis. Inhibition of atherogenesis by probucol indeed has been observed in genetically hyperlipidemic rabbits. Thus, probucol may be beneficial for prevention of atherosclerosis beyond its effects on serum lipoprotein levels.

DOSAGE

Probucol is available in 250 mg and 500 mg tablets. The usual dosage is 500 mg twice daily. The drug accumulates in the adipose tissue of the body, and it disappears from the circulation only very slowly after it has been discontinued.

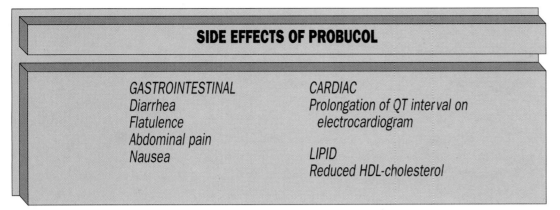

Fig. 4.40 Side effects of probucol.

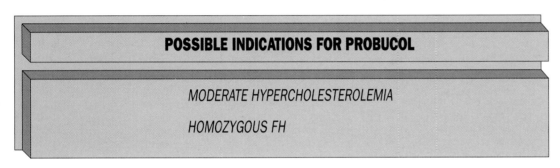

Fig. 4.41 Possible indications for probucol.

SIDE EFFECTS

In general, probucol is well tolerated by most patients, and side effects usually are minimal (Fig. 4.40). Most side effects are limited to the gastrointestinal tract. Typical complaints are diarrhea, flatulence, abdominal pain, and nausea. Moreover, the drug can cause prolongation of the QT interval on electrocardiogram and, therefore, is contraindicated if patients have cardiac arrhythmias related to or accompanied by changes in the QT interval. Also, probucol should not be given concomitantly with other drugs that alter the QT interval. Finally, probucol lowers the HDL-cholesterol fraction. Whether this offsets the beneficial effect in LDL lowering is not known. It must be noted, in addition, that the long-term safety of probucol has not been documented in a clinical trial.

INDICATIONS

Probucol is one drug among several that might be used for treatment of primary moderate hypercholesterolemia (Fig. 4.41). Generally, it causes a lowering of LDL-cholesterol of approximately 15%, and this action combined with dietary therapy should reduce LDL-cholesterol levels to the desirable range in many patients. Since probucol has not been shown to reduce the risk for CHD in a major clinical trial, it cannot be considered a drug of first choice. Moreover, its lowering of HDL-choles-

terol levels can be considered a theoretical drawback. On the other hand, the drug protects LDL from oxidation, which may be an advantage. Use of probucol in combination with a bile acid sequestrant has been shown to enhance the LDL-lowering action.

Probucol apparently lowers cholesterol levels in patients with homozygous FH, and it can even cause regression of xanthomas in some patients of this type. Although it cannot be considered the only mode of therapy in this disorder, it might be used as an adjunct with more effective cholesterol-lowering drugs.

DRUG THERAPY OF VARIOUS HYPERLIPIDEMIAS

FAMILIAL HYPERCHOLESTEROLEMIA

The usual form of familial hypercholesterolemia (FH) is heterozygous, indicating that affected individuals have inherited only one functional gene for synthesis of LDL receptors (see Figs. 2.25–2.27). As a result of this defect, LDL-receptor activity is decreased, and LDL-cholesterol levels are approximately twice normal. As with other forms of hyperlipidemia, dietary therapy alone is the first mode of treatment. In general, however, dietary therapy is inadequate to lower LDL levels to within the normal range, and concomitant drug therapy is required. Thus, in patients with heterozygous FH, a six-month trial

of dietary therapy is not necessary before they can be started on drug therapy. This is not to say that dietary modification is not beneficial; heterozygous FH patients often respond to dietary therapy with significant reductions in LDL levels, and consequently it should always be employed along with drug treatment.

The drug of first choice for heterozygous FH is a bile acid sequestrant. Patients should be urged to take the maximal tolerated dose of sequestrant. With proper instruction and guidance, most patients can tolerate 16 g of cholestyramine or 20 g of colestipol daily, and some can adjust to even higher doses. It may be helpful to start bile acid sequestrants at relatively small doses and then gradually but progressively increase the dose. Yet, despite taking relatively high doses of drugs and achieving significant reductions in LDL-cholesterol levels, most FH heterozygotes have LDL values that usually remain well above desirable, and consideration must be given to use of another drug in combination.

One drug combination—a bile acid sequestrant plus nicotinic acid—has been tested extensively. This regimen not only lowers LDL-cholesterol concentrations, but it also raises HDL-cholesterol levels. Reductions in LDL-cholesterol of 35% to 40% are typical. LDL-receptor activity is increased by the bile acid sequestrant, while nicotinic acid

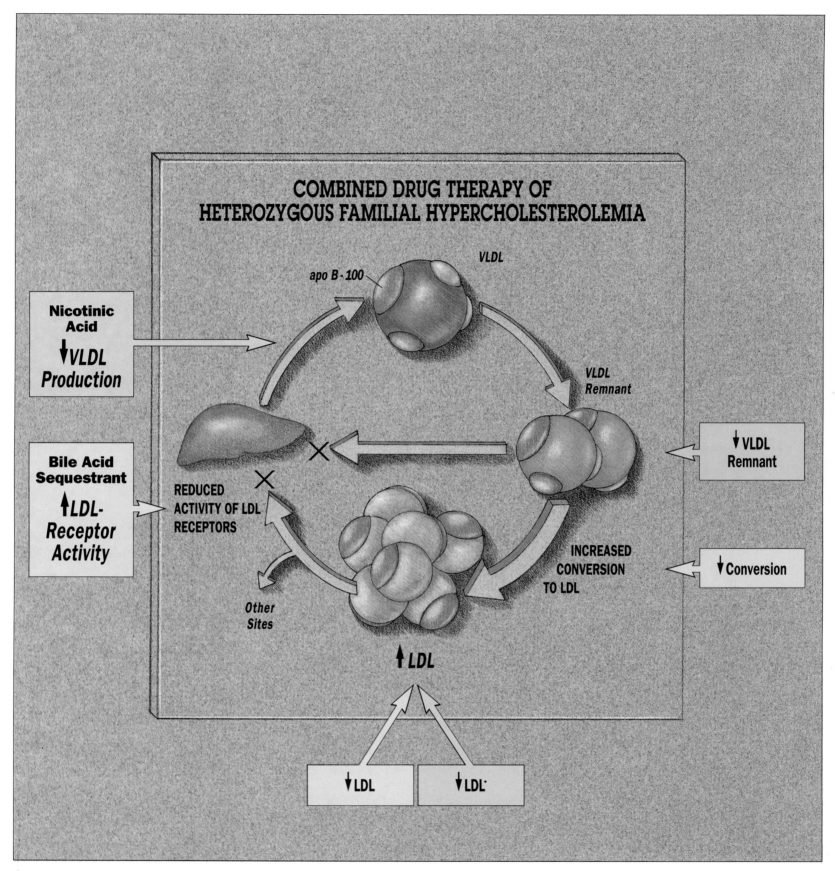

Fig. 4.42 Major actions of combined therapy with a bile acid sequestrant and nicotinic acid on the lipoprotein abnormalities found in heterozygous FH (see also Figs. 4.6, 4.16).

inhibits hepatic production of lipoproteins. The combination, therefore, lowers LDL levels in two ways, by decreasing input of lipoproteins (nicotinic acid) and enhancing their clearance (seques-

trants) (Fig. 4.42). Another potent drug combination is a bile acid sequestrant plus a HMG-CoA reductase inhibitor (Fig. 4.43). Both of these drugs enhance the activity of LDL receptors by decreas-

ing hepatic content of cholesterol. Bile acid sequestrants promote conversion of cholesterol into bile acids, whereas HMG-CoA reductase inhibitors block the formation of cholesterol. This drug com-

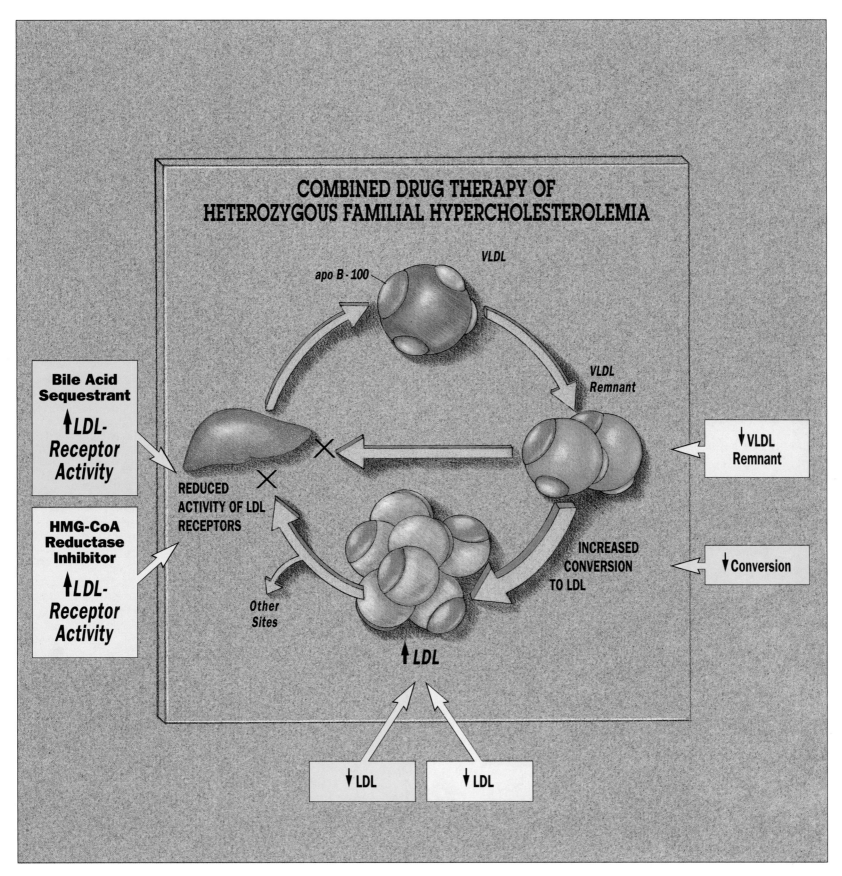

Fig. 4.43 Major actions of combined therapy with a bile acid sequestrant and a HMG-CoA reductase inhibitor on the lipoprotein abnormalities found in heterozygous FH (see also Figs. 4.6, 4.23).

bination produces a marked reduction in hepatic cholesterol content and doubly stimulates the synthesis of LDL receptors. In patients with heterozygous FH, LDL-cholesterol levels are decreased by 45% to 60%; in other words, they are reduced to near the desirable level.

In rare cases, patients inherit two nonfunctional genes for LDL-receptor synthesis, one from each parent. These patients thus have homozygous FH and severe elevations of LDL-cholesterol; they have virtually no normal LDL receptors. Therapeutic approaches for homozygous FH are outlined in Figure

TREATMENT OF HOMOZYGOUS FAMILIAL HYPERCHOLESTEROLEMIA

DRUG THERAPY*	LDL PLASMAPHERESIS
Nicotinic acid	
Probucol	LIVER TRANSPLANT

*Bile acid sequestrants and HMG-CoA reductase inhibitors have no effect.

Fig. 4.44 Treatment of homozygous FH.

ETIOLOGY OF PRIMARY SEVERE HYPERCHOLESTEROLEMIA

NONCLASSICAL HETEROZYGOUS FH

METABOLIC SUPPRESSION OF LDL-RECEPTOR ACTIVITY

FAMILIAL DEFECTIVE APOLIPOPROTEIN B-100

Fig. 4.45 Etiology of primary severe hypercholesterolemia.

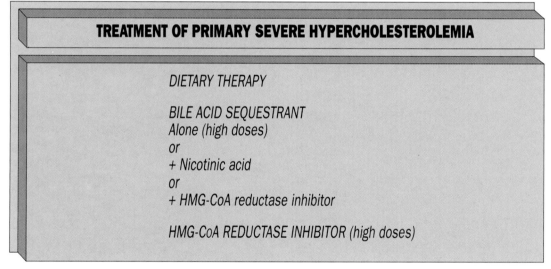

TREATMENT OF PRIMARY SEVERE HYPERCHOLESTEROLEMIA

DIETARY THERAPY

BILE ACID SEQUESTRANT
Alone (high doses)
or
+ Nicotinic acid
or
+ HMG-CoA reductase inhibitor

HMG-CoA REDUCTASE INHIBITOR (high doses)

Fig. 4.46 Treatment of primary severe hypercholesterolemia.

4.44. Drugs that act mainly by increasing the activity of LDL receptors, i.e., bile acid sequestrants and HMG-CoA reductase inhibitors, have essentially no effect on LDL-cholesterol concentrations. In contrast, nicotinic acid, which inhibits the formation of lipoproteins, causes a lowering of LDL levels, but the degree of reduction is not adequate to achieve therapeutic success. The drug probucol also modestly reduces LDL-cholesterol levels in FH homozygotes, possibly by increasing nonreceptor clearance of LDL. Nonpharmacologic approaches also have been employed for therapy of homozygous FH. Excess LDL in circulation can be temporarily reduced by plasmapheresis or by extracorporeal removal of LDL by LDL-binding columns. This latter approach is becoming standard therapy for FH homozygotes. Another form of therapy is liver transplantation. By replacing the patient's liver with the liver from a normal person, a normal complement of hepatic LDL receptors can be restored. This latter technique proved successful for treatment of severe hypercholesterolemia in at least one patient with homozygous FH.

PRIMARY SEVERE HYPERCHOLESTEROLEMIA

Many patients with severe hypercholesterolemia do not have classical FH; i.e., they do not exhibit tendon xanthomas, or have a strong family history of hypercholesterolemia and premature CHD. Such patients, nonetheless, can have cholesterol levels near the range typically observed in patients with heterozygous FH. Most of these patients appear to have retarded clearance of serum LDL, which may be the result of several abnormalities—nonclassical heterozygous FH, regulatory defects with metabolic suppression of LDL-receptor synthesis, or familial defective apolipoprotein B-100 (see Fig. 2.29) (Fig. 4.45). Treatment of severe nonfamilial hypercholesterolemia is similar to that of heterozygous FH (Fig. 4.46). Baseline therapy should include appropriate diet modification, and bile acid sequestrants are the drug of first choice.

TREATMENT OF PRIMARY MODERATE HYPERCHOLESTEROLEMIA

STEPWISE APPROACH
Dietary therapy
Bile acid sequestrant (low to moderate dose)
Bile acid sequestrant
+ HMG-CoA reductase inhibitor (low dose)

ALTERNATIVE DRUGS
Nicotinic acid
HMG-CoA reductase inhibitor
Gemfibrozil
Probucol

Fig. 4.47 Treatment of primary moderate hypercholesterolemia.

If the combination of dietary and sequestrant therapy does not "normalize" LDL levels, consideration can be given to use of a second drug, either nicotinic acid or a HMG-CoA reductase inhibitor (see Figs. 4.42, 4.43). Some patients can be treated satisfactorily with relatively high doses of reductase inhibitor alone, although the danger of side effects is increased (see Figs. 4.24, 4.25).

PRIMARY MODERATE HYPERCHOLESTEROLEMIA

The recommended approach to this condition, outlined in Figure 4.47, is a stepwise approach. Moderate elevations of LDL-cholesterol in many patients can be controlled adequately with dietary therapy. Still, for those with levels approaching the severely elevated range, drug therapy may be required. In such cases, bile acid sequestrants are first-line therapy after diet modification. Often LDL levels can be reduced adequately with the combination of dietary modification and low doses of a bile acid sequestrant; some cases, however, require moderate doses of a sequestrant. An alternate drug that can be used for this condition is nicotinic acid, but the usefulness of this drug is limited because of the common occurrence of side effects. Indications for HMG-CoA reductase inhibitors for primary moderate hypercholesterolemia have not been fully defined. One approach is to add a small dose of HMG-CoA reductase inhibitor to a bile acid sequestrant. Since long-term side effects of HMG-CoA reductase inhibitors have not been ruled out, it may be prudent to withhold higher doses of these agents in patients with moderate hypercholesterolemia who are not otherwise at high risk for CHD. On the other hand, if a patient is at high risk because of other factors, use of a HMG-CoA reductase inhibitor probably can be justified. Yet another approach is to use gemfibrozil combined with dietary therapy. In the Helsinki Heart Study, this drug significantly reduced the risk for CHD in patients with moderate hypercholesterolemia. Finally, probucol can be used for treatment of moderate hypercholesterolemia, but its best use may be as a second agent in combination with a bile acid sequestrant.

PRIMARY MIXED HYPERLIPIDEMIA

Increased serum levels of both cholesterol (over 240 mg/dl) and triglyceride (250 to 500 mg/dl) appear to be accompanied by an especially high risk for CHD. This pattern of dyslipidemia can have several causes. One of these is the genetic disorder called *familial combined hyperlipidemia*, a condition characterized by multiple lipoprotein phenotypes in a single family (see Fig. 2.32). One clinical manifestation of familial combined hyperlipidemia is mixed hyperlipidemia, which often presents as type IIB HLP. Lipid-lowering drug therapy can be justified in many patients with primary mixed hyperlipidemia; several approaches can be taken.

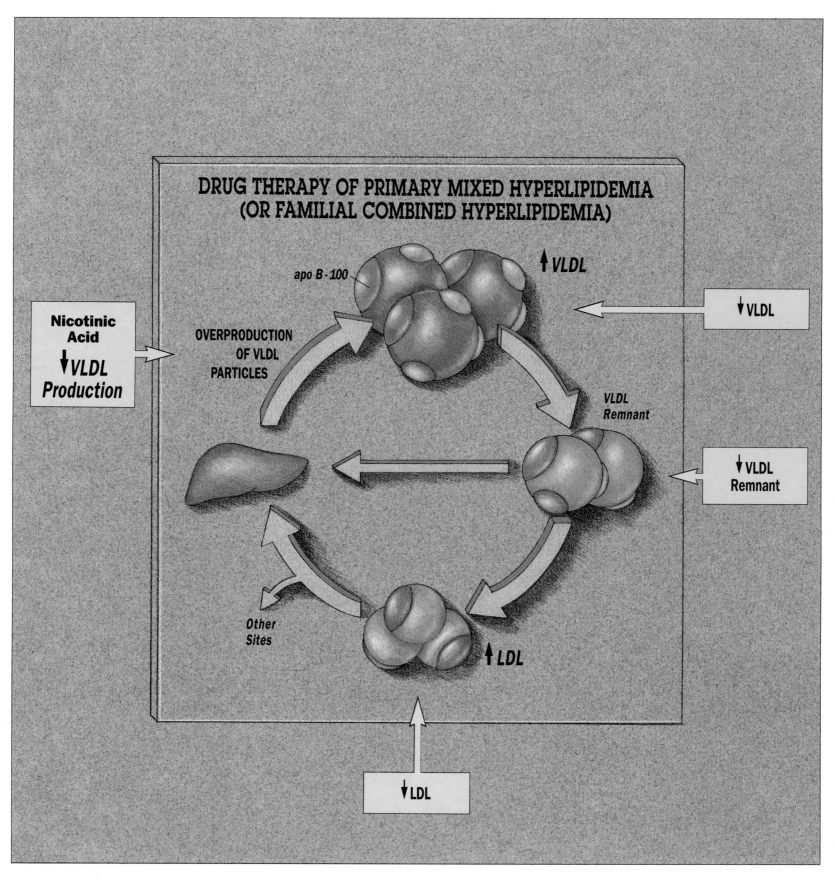

Fig. 4.48 Major actions of nicotinic acid therapy on the disordered metabolic pathways found in primary mixed hyperlipidemia (or familial combined hyperlipidemia) (see also Fig. 4.16).

Theoretically, the drug of first choice for treatment of familial combined hyperlipidemia is nicotinic acid, because it acts to reduce the formation of lipoproteins by the liver, reversing an important underlying cause of the condition (see Figs. 2.33, 2.34) (Fig. 4.48). If patients with familial combined hyperlipidemia can tolerate nicotinic acid, this drug alone may be sufficient to correct the several lipoprotein abnormalities that occur in this disorder. An alternative to nicotinic acid in patients with mixed hyperlipidemia is gemfibrozil. In the Helsinki Heart Study, this drug appeared to reduce the risk for CHD in patients with one form of mixed hyperlipidemia, namely, type IIB HLP.

Still another drug that can be used in treatment of primary mixed hyperlipidemia is a HMG-CoA reductase in-

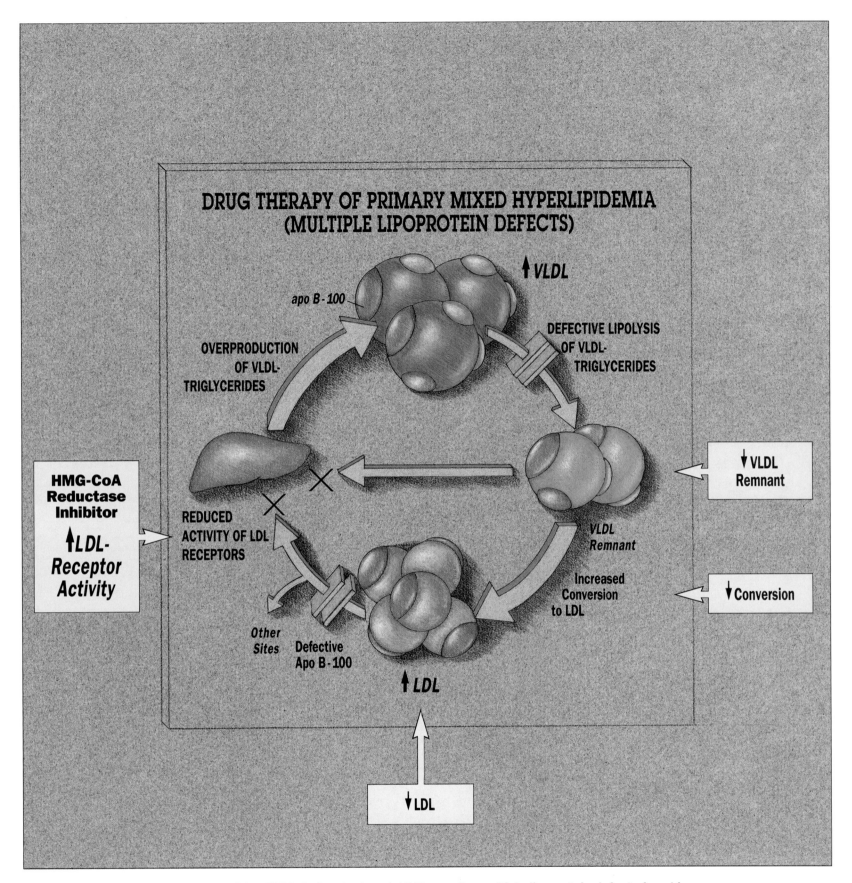

Fig. 4.49 Major actions of therapy with a HMG-CoA reductase inhibitor on the multiple lipoprotein defects found in primary mixed hyperlipidemia (see also Fig. 4.23).

hibitor (Fig. 4.49). Drugs of this class lower serum concentrations of both VLDL and LDL (see Fig. 4.23), and thus will improve the abnormal lipoprotein pattern in individuals with mixed hyperlipidemia. It must be noted, however, that reductase inhibitors usually do not appreciably raise HDL-cholesterol concentrations in most patients. Nonetheless, because of their efficacy in cholesterol lowering, HMG-CoA reductase inhibitors can be considered for treatment of familial combined hyperlipidemia if previously discussed drugs do not produce an adequate response.

Elevations of both serum cholesterol and triglycerides often can be treated more effectively with combined drug therapy than with monotherapy. The combination of nicotinic acid and a bile

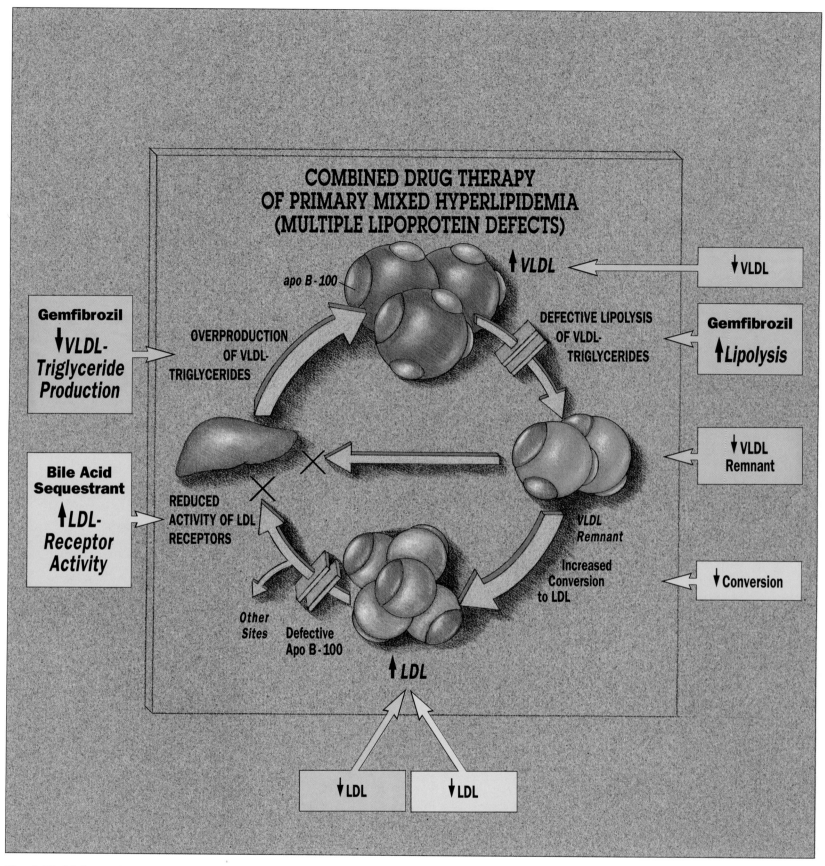

Fig. 4.50 Major actions of combined therapy with a bile acid sequestrant and gemfibrozil on the multiple lipoprotein defects found in primary mixed hyperlipidemia (see also Figs. 4.6, 4.28, 4.29).

acid sequestrant produces enhanced lowering of total-cholesterol and LDL-cholesterol levels. If nicotinic acid cannot be tolerated, gemfibrozil (or another fibric acid) can be used in combination with a bile acid sequestrant (Fig. 4.50). Gemfibrozil plus lovastatin has proved to be highly effective for treatment of familial combined hyperlipidemia, but this drug regimen carries a relatively high risk for severe myopathy. The same danger apparently is present with the combination of nicotinic acid and a HMG-CoA reductase inhibitor.

In the minds of many investigators, familial combined hyperlipidemia represents a disorder characterized by primary overproduction of lipoproteins by the liver (see Fig. 2.33). However, it is possible that multiple primary lipoprotein defects can be inherited simultane-

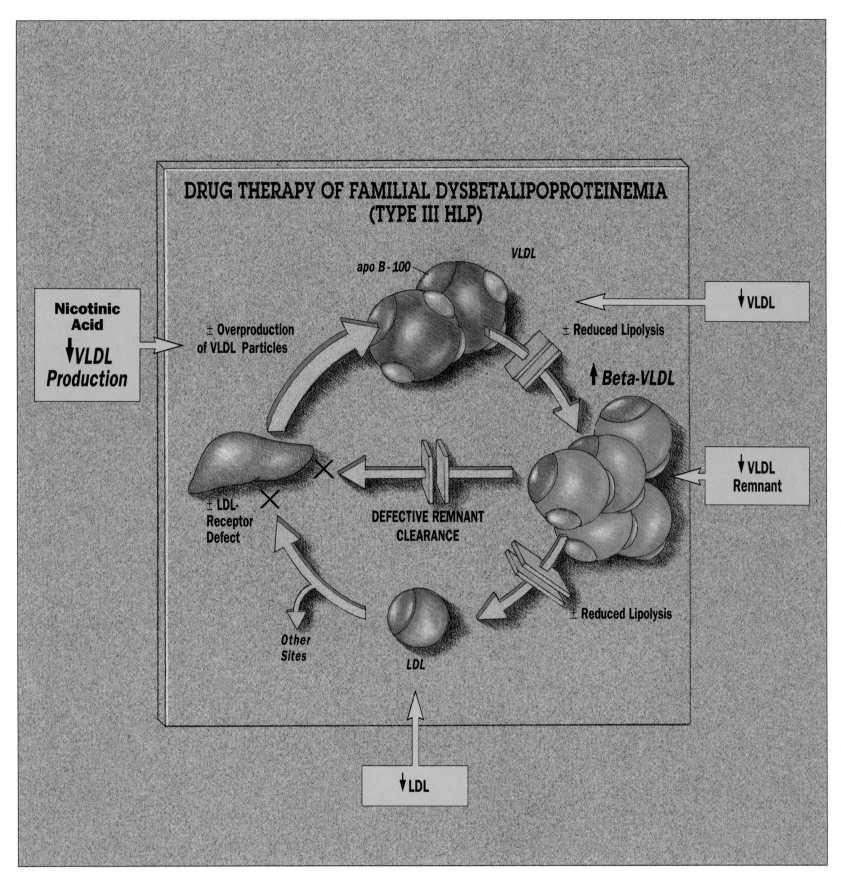

Fig. 4.51 Major actions of nicotinic acid therapy on the disordered metabolic pathways found in familial dysbeta-lipoproteinemia (type III HLP) (see also Fig. 4.16).

ously in a single family (see Fig. 2.34). Regardless of the underlying cause, the general approach to therapy of mixed hyperlipidemia probably should depend on the pattern of dyslipidemia in a given individual rather than a postulated etiology.

FAMILIAL DYSBETALIPOPROTEINEMIA (TYPE III HLP)

This disorder is characterized by an increase in both cholesterol and triglycerides in the VLDL fraction. An abnormal type of VLDL, called beta-VLDL, is present, resulting from a defect in the structure of apolipoprotein E (see Fig. 2.19). Patients with type III HLP are at increased risk for CHD. Often the excess beta-VLDL can be eliminated by dietary means—weight loss and reduction in intakes of saturated fatty acids

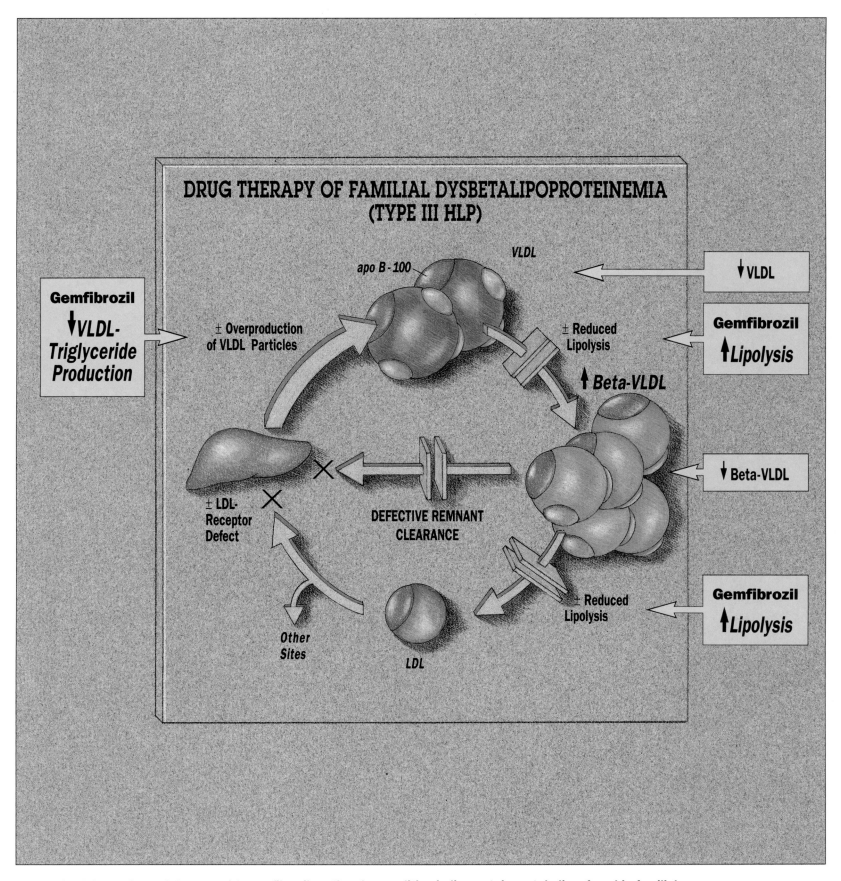

Fig. 4.52 Major actions of therapy with gemfibrozil on the abnormalities in lipoprotein metabolism found in familial dysbetalipoproteinemia (type III HLP) (see also Figs. 4.28, 4.29).

and cholesterol. In many cases, however, it is necessary to use drug therapy. Nicotinic acid is considered the drug of choice, because it reduces beta-VLDL by decreasing the input of VLDL (Fig. 4.51; *see previous page*). If nicotinic acid cannot be tolerated, gemfibrozil is a good alternative because it reduces formation of VLDL and promotes its catabolism (Fig. 4.52). Finally, a HMG-CoA reductase inhibitor can be effective when the cholesterol level is markedly elevated. A reductase inhibitor promotes the clearance of beta-VLDL by the liver (Fig. 4.53). In most patients with type III HLP, lipid levels can be normalized by the combination of dietary therapy and one of the drugs mentioned above.

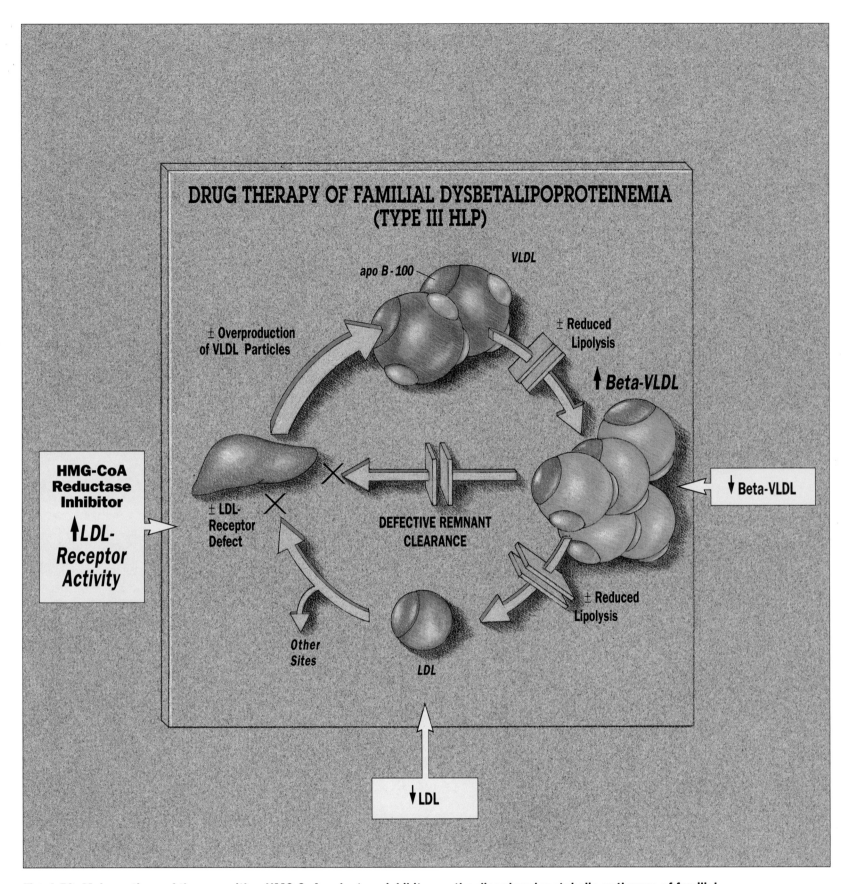

Fig. 4.53 Major actions of therapy with a HMG-CoA reductase inhibitor on the disordered metabolic pathways of familial dysbetalipoproteinemia (type III HLP) (see also Fig. 4.23).

MODERATE HYPERTRIGLYCERIDEMIA (TYPE IV HLP)

Moderate hypertriglyceridemia (serum triglycerides in the range of 250 to 500 mg/dl) often has a dietary basis or is secondary to another disease. Obesity appears to be the most common cause, and alcohol can be a contributing factor. Weight reduction and avoidance of alcohol thus can be considered first-line therapy for moderate hypertriglyceridemia. Drug therapy should be reserved for individuals in whom risk for CHD is high due to other factors, e.g., previous atherosclerotic disease, strong family history of CHD, persistent smoking, diabetes mellitus, and poorly controlled hypertension (Fig. 4.54; *see next page*). Three different drugs can be employed for treatment in these cases.

**INDICATIONS FOR DRUG THERAPY OF
MODERATE HYPERTRIGLYCERIDEMIA (TYPE IV HLP)**

HIGH-RISK PATIENTS
History of CHD or other atherosclerotic disease
Family history of premature CHD
Persistent smoking
Diabetes mellitus
Poorly controlled hypertension

Fig. 4.54 Indications for drug therapy of moderate hypertriglyceridemia (type IV HLP).

Nicotinic acid is the drug of choice except in patients with diabetes in whom this drug can worsen hyperglycemia (Fig. 4.55). Gemfibrozil also will normalize triglyceride levels in most patients (Fig. 4.56; *see page 4.42*); at the same time, however, LDL-cholesterol levels may rise. Whether lowering triglyceride containing lipoproteins by drug therapy will reduce the risk for CHD in patients with moderate hypertriglyceridemia has not been determined.

SEVERE HYPERTRIGLYCERIDEMIA (TYPE V HLP)

Marked elevations of serum triglycerides usually are accompanied by increases in both VLDL and chylomicrons (type V HLP) (see Fig. 2.21). Such patients usually have a genetic defect in clearance of triglyceride-rich lipoproteins and overproduction of VLDL from secondary causes (e.g., obesity, excess alcohol intake, or diabetes mellitus). The immediate concern for patients with this condition is the development of acute pancreatitis, which may occur when triglyceride concentrations exceed 1500 mg/dl. Many patients with type V HLP probably are at increased risk for CHD, but therapeutic priority must be given to reducing the chances for acute pancreatitis. Both dietary modification and use of triglyceride-lowering drugs may be required. Dietary therapy includes weight reduction, restriction of alcohol intake, and decreased consumption of dietary fat. Diabetic patients may require better control of hyperglycemia to lower triglyceride levels. If these measures do not bring triglyceride concentrations to below 1000 mg/dl, and preferably to below 500 mg/dl, triglyceride-lowering agents may be required. Nicotinic acid can be tried first, but if it is not well tolerated, gemfibrozil should be employed (Fig. 4.57; *see page 4.43*). In most instances, gemfibrozil reduces triglyceride concentrations to a level that eliminates the danger for acute pancreatitis. However, triglyceride levels frequently remain moderately elevated in spite of drug therapy, and normalization of serum triglycerides is extremely difficult, if not impossible.

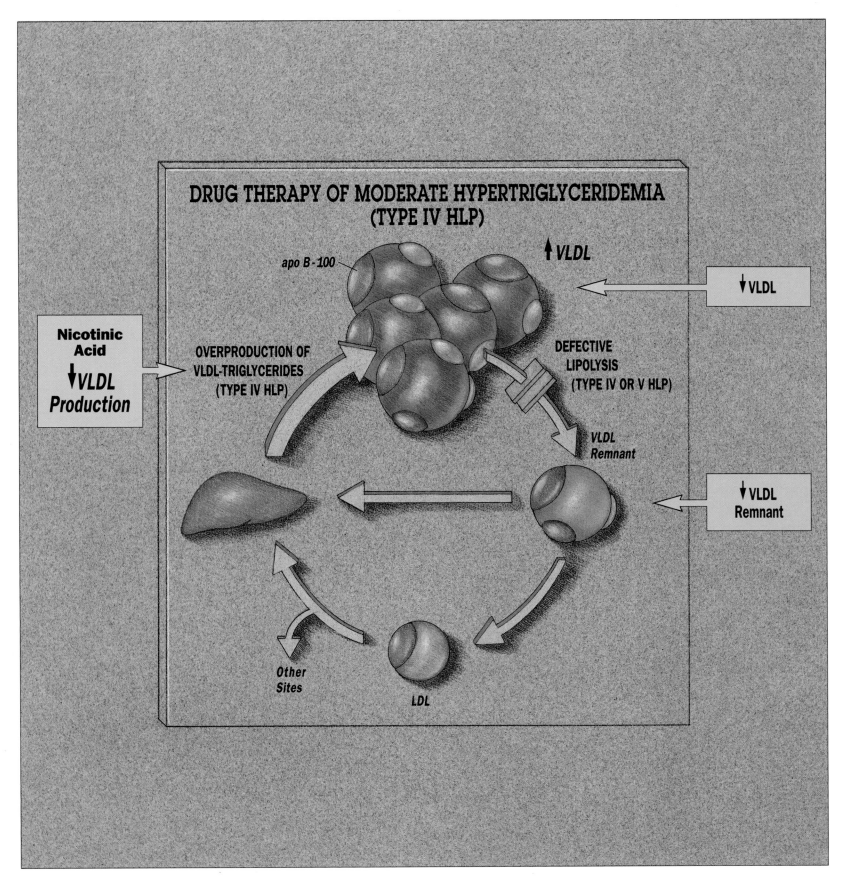

Fig. 4.55 Major actions of nicotinic acid therapy on the abnormalities in lipoprotein metabolism found in moderate hypertriglyceridemia (type IV HLP) (see also Fig. 4.16).

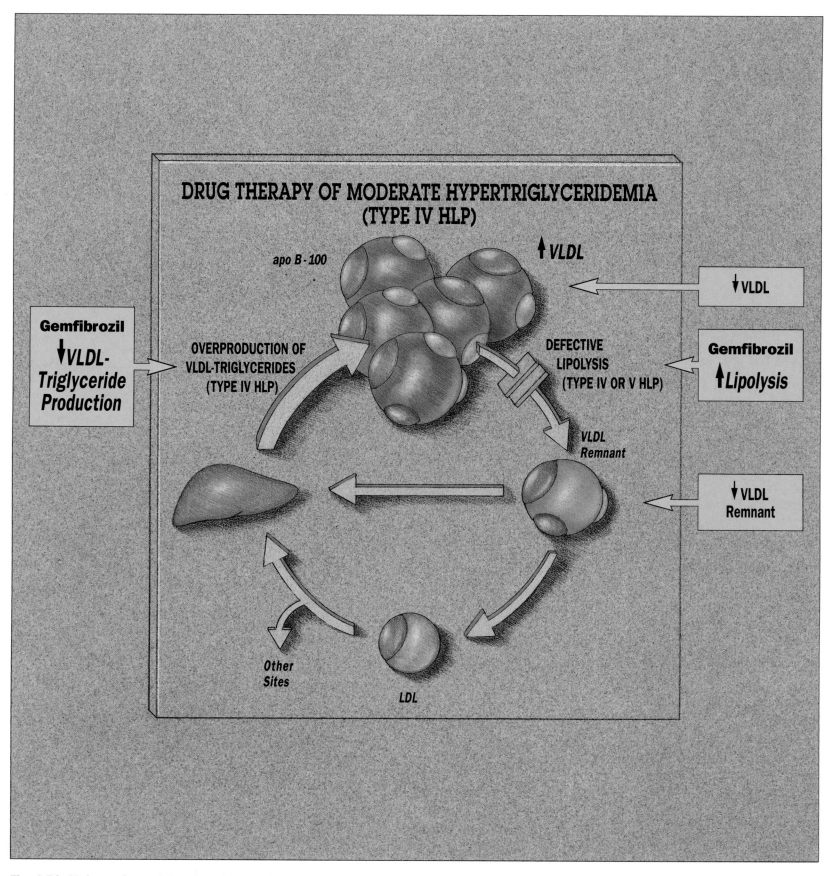

Fig. 4.56 Major actions of therapy with gemfibrozil on the lipoprotein abnormalities found in moderate hypertriglyceridemia (type IV HLP) (see also Fig 4.28).

HYPOALPHALIPOPROTEINEMIA

In many cases, a low concentration of HDL-cholesterol is the result of external factors (e.g., obesity, lack of exercise, cigarette smoking, and use of androgenic and related steroids) (see Fig. 2.10). These factors should be modified first in patients with low HDL. When a low HDL-cholesterol concentration occurs in the presence of another dyslipidemia, it may be reasonable to turn to drug therapy. This is particularly true when a low HDL concentration is combined with elevated LDL-cholesterol. The presence of a low HDL-cholesterol favors use of nicotinic acid or gemfibrozil, because either of these agents can raise

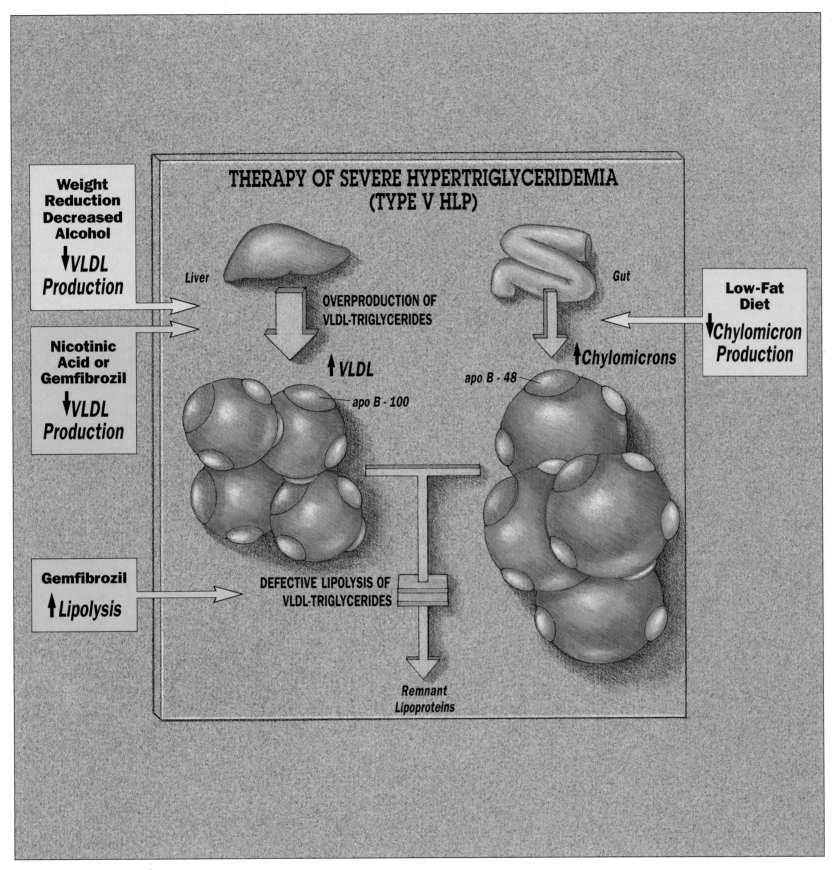

Fig. 4.57 Major actions of dietary modification and drug therapy with either nicotinic acid or gemfibrozil on the lipoprotein abnormalities characterizing severe hypertriglyceridemia (type V HLP) (see also Figs. 4.16, 4.21).

the HDL level. Enhanced LDL lowering can be obtained by combining either of these drugs with a bile acid sequestrant, but not with lovastatin because of the high risk for myopathy. Drug treatment of isolated low HDL-cholesterol, in the absence of elevation of other lipoproteins, is controversial. Recently, lovastatin has been shown to produce a marked reduction of LDL-C/HDL-C ratios in normolipidemic patients with low HDL, but use of lovastatin for this purpose probably should be reserved for high-risk patients. With lovastatin, the decrease in the LDL-C/HDL-C ratio is due almost entirely to a decrease in the LDL fraction, whereas HDL-cholesterol is increased only modestly.

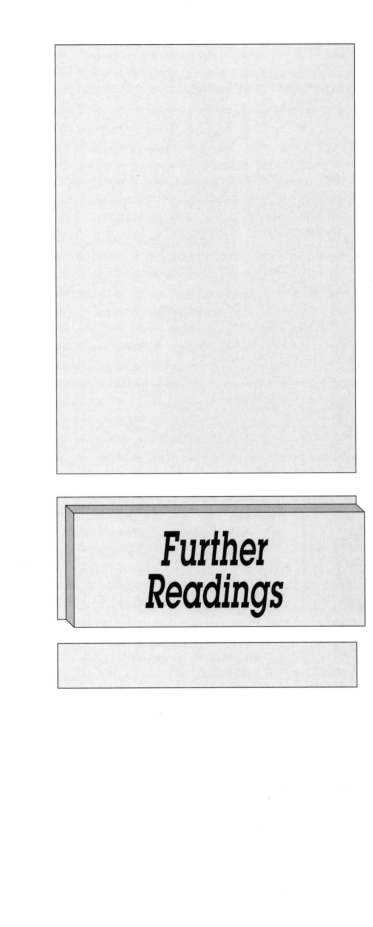

Further Readings

Unit One

Cholesterol, Atherosclerosis and Coronary Heart Disease

Abbott RD, Wilson PWF, Kannel WB, et al: High density lipoprotein cholesterol, total cholesterol screening, and myocardial infarction. *Arteriosclerosis* 8:207–211, 1988.

Brown MS, Goldstein JL: Receptor-mediated pathway for cholesterol homeostasis. *Science* 232:34–47, 1986.

Brown MS, Goldstein JL: How LDL receptors influence cholesterol and atherosclerosis. *Scientific American* 251(5):58–66, 1984.

Brown MS, Goldstein JL: Lipoprotein metabolism in the macrophage. *Annu Rev Biochem* 52:223, 1983.

Brown MS, Goldstein JL: Lipoprotein receptors in the liver: control signals for plasma cholesterol traffic. *J Clin Invest* 72:743–747, 1983.

Brown MS, Goldstein JL: Receptor-mediated control of cholesterol metabolism. *Science* 191:150–154, 1976.

Brown MS, Kovanen PT, Goldstein JL: Regulation of plasma cholesterol by lipoprotein receptors. *Science* 212:628–635, 1981.

Castelli WP, Doyle JT, Gordon T, et al: HDL cholesterol and other lipids in coronary heart disease: the cooperative lipoprotein phenotyping study. *Circulation* 55:767–772, 1977.

Consensus Development Conference. Lowering blood cholesterol to prevent heart disease. *JAMA* 253:2080–2086, 1985.

Cotran RS, Munro JM: Pathogenesis of atherosclerosis: recent concepts, in Grundy SM, Bearn AG (eds): *The Role of Cholesterol in Atherosclerosis: New Therapeutic Opportunities*. Hanley and Belfus, Philadelphia, 1988, pp 5–21.

Eder HA, Gidex LI: The clinical significance of plasma high density lipoproteins. *Med Clin North Am* 66:431, 1982.

Eisenberg S: High density lipoprotein metabolism. *J Lipid Res* 25:1017, 1984.

Fielding CJ, Fielding PE: Cholesterol transport between cells and body fluids: role of plasma lipoproteins and plasma cholesterol esterification system. *Med Clin North Am* 66:363–373, 1982.

Fogelman AM, Shechter I, Seager J, et al: Malondialdehyde altertion of LDL leads to cholesterol ester accumulation in human monocyte-macrophages. *Proc Natl Acad Sci USA* 7:221, 1980.

Goldbourt V, Holtzman E, Neufeld HN: Total and high density lipoprotein cholesterol in the serum and risk of mortality: evidence of a threshold effect. *Br Med J* 290:1239–1243, 1985.

Goldstein JL, Brown MS: The low-density lipoprotein pathway and its relation to atherosclerosis. *Annu Rev Biochem* 46:897–930. 1977.

Goldstein JL, Ho YK, Basu SK: A binding site on macrophages that mediates the uptake and degradation of acetylated low density lipoprotein. *Proc Natl Acad Sci USA* 76:333, 1979.

Gordon T, Castelli WP, Hjortland MC, et al: High density lipoprotein as a protective factor against coronary heart disease: the Framingham study. *Am J Med* 62:707–714, 1977.

Gotto AM Jr, Pownall HR, Havel RJ: Introduction to the plasma lipoproteins. *Methods Enzymol* 128:3, 1986.

Grundy SM: Cholesterol and coronary heart disease: a new era. *JAMA* 256:2849–2858, 1986.

Grundy SM: Atherosclerosis: pathology, pathogenesis, and role of risk factors. *Disease-a-Month* 29(9):1–58, 1983.

Harker LA: Platlets, endothelial injury, and atherosclerosis, in Steinberg D, Olefsky JM (eds): *Hypercholesterolemia and Atherosclerosis: Pathogenesis and Prevention*. Churchill Livingstone, New York, 1987, pp 25–52.

Kannel WB, Castelli WP, Gordon T: Cholesterol in the prediction of atherosclerotic disease: new perspectives in the Framingham study. *Ann Intern Med* 90:85–91, 1979.

Kannel WB, Castelli W, Gordon T, et al: Serum cholesterol, lipoproteins, and risk of coronary heart disease: the Framingham study. *Ann Intern Med* 74:1–12, 1971.

Kannel WB, Neaton JD, Wentworth D, et al: Overall and CHD mortality rates in relation to major risk factors in 325,348 men screened for the MRFIT. *Am Heart J* 112:825–836, 1986.

Keys A (ed): Coronary heart disease in seven countries. *Circulation* 41(suppl 1):1–211, 1970.

Krauss RM: Regulation of high density lipoprotein levels. *Med Clin North Am* 66:403–430, 1982.

Lerner DJ, Kannel WB: Patterns of coronary heart disease morbidity and mortality in the sexes: a twenty-six year follow-up of the Framingham population. *Am Heart J* 111:383–390, 1986.

Lowering blood cholesterol to prevent heart disease. *JAMA* 253:2080–2086, 1985.

Mahley RW: Apolipoprotein E: cholesterol transport protein with expanding role in cell biology. *Science* 240:622, 1988.

Mahley RW: Atherogenic hyperlipoproteinemia: the cellular and molecular biology of plasma lipoproteins altered by dietary fat and cholesterol. *Med Clin North Am* 66:375–402, 1982.

Martin MJ, Hulley SB, Browner WS, et al: Serum cholesterol, blood pressure, and mortality: implications from a cohort of 361,662 men. *Lancet* 2:933–936, 1986.

McGill HC Jr: Persistent problems in the pathogenesis of atherosclerosis. *Arteriosclerosis* 4:443, 1984.

Miller GJ, Miller NE: Plasma high density lipoprotein concentration and development of ischaemic heart disease. *Lancet* 1:16–19, 1975.

Relationship of blood pressure, serum cholesterol, smoking habit, relative weight and ECG abnormalities to incidence of major coronary events: final report of the Pooling Project Research Group. *J Chronic Dis* 31:201–306, 1978.

Ross R: The pathogenesis of atherosclerosis—an update. *N Engl J Med* 314:488–500, 1986.

Ross R, Glomset JA: The pathogenesis of atherosclerosis. *N Engl J Med* 295:369–377, 420–425, 1976.

Schaefer EJ, Eisenberg S, Levy RI: Lipoprotein apoprotein metabolism. *J Lipid Res* 19:667–687, 1978.

Solberg LA, Strong JP: Risk factors and atherosclerotic lesions: a review of autopsy studies. *Arteriosclerosis* 3:187–198, 1983.

Stamler J, Wentworth D, Neaton J: Is the relationship between serum cholesterol and risk of death from CHD continuous and graded? *JAMA* 256:2823–2828, 1986.

Stary HC: Evolution of atherosclerotic plaques in coronary arteries of young adults. *Arteriosclerosis* 3:471, 1983.

Steinberg D: Current theories of the pathogenesis of atherosclerosis, in Steinberg D, Olefsky JM (eds): *Hypercholesterolemia and Atherosclerosis: Pathogenesis and Prevention*. Churchill Livingstone, New York, 1987, pp 5–23.

Steinberg D: Lipoproteins and atherosclerosis: a look back and a look ahead. *Arteriosclerosis* 3:283–301, 1983.

Steinberg D, Parthasarathy S, Carew TE, et al: Beyond cholesterol: modifications of low-density lipoprotein that increase its atherogenicity. *N Eng J Med* 320:915–923, 1989.

van Tol A: Reverse cholesterol transport, in Steinmetz A, Schneider HJ (eds): *Cholesterol Transport Systems and Their Relation to Atherosclerosis*. Springer-Verlag, Berlin Heidelberg, 1989, pp 85–88.

Zilversmit DB: Atherogenesis: a postprandial phenomenon. *Circulation* 60:473, 1979.

Unit Two

Classification of Lipid Disorders

Abrams JJ, Ginsberg H, Grundy SM: Metabolism of cholesterol and plasma triglycerides in nonketotic diabetes mellitus. *Diabetes* 31:903–910, 1982.

Appel GB, Blum CB, Chien S, et al: The hyperlipidemia of the nephrotic syndrome: relation to plasma albumin concentration, oncotic pressure and viscosity. *N Engl J Med* 312:1544, 1985.

Barrett-Connor E, Grundy SM, Holdbrook MJ: Plasma lipids and diabetes mellitus in an adult community. *Am J Epidemiol* 115:657–663, 1982.

Bilheimer DW, Stone NJ, Grundy SM: Metabolic studies in familial hypercholesterolemia: evidence for a gene-dosage effect in vivo. *J Clin Invest* 64:524–533, 1979.

Brown MS, Goldstein JL, Fredrickson DS: Familial type 3 hyperlipoproteinemia (dysbetalipoproteinemia), in: Stanbury JB, Wyngaarden JB, Fredrickson DS, et al (eds): *The Metabolic Basis of Inherited Disease*, 5th ed. McGraw-Hill, New York, 1983, p 655.

Brunzell JD, Bierman EL: Chylomicronemia syndrome: interaction of genetic and acquired hypertriglyceridemia. *Med Clin North Am* 66:455, 1982.

Brunzell JD, Schrott HG, Motulsky AG, et al: Myocardial infarction in the familial forms of hypertriglyceridemia. *Metabolism* 25:313–320, 1976.

Brunzell JD, Hazzard WR, Motulsky AG, et al: Evidence for diabetes mellitus and genetic forms of hypertriglyceridemia as separate entities. *Metabolism* 24:1115, 1975.

Carlson LA, Bottinger LE, Ahfeldt P-E: Risk factors for myocardial infarction in the Stockholm prospective study: a 14-year follow-up focusing on the role of plasma triglyceride and cholesterol. *Acta Med Scand* 206:351–360, 1979.

Castelli WP: The triglyceride issue: a view from Framingham. *Am Heart J* 112:432–437, 1986.

Chait A, Albers JJ, Brunzell JD: Very low density lipoprotein overproduction in genetic forms of hypertriglyceridaemia. *Eur J Clin Invest* 10:17–22, 1980.

Consensus Development Conference. Treatment of hypertriglyceridemia. *JAMA* 251:1196–1200, 1984.

Fredrickson DS, Levy RI, Lees RS: Fat transport in lipoproteins—an integrated approach to mechanisms and disorders. *N Engl J Med* 276:32, 94, 148, 215, 273, 1967.

Glomset JA: The plasma lecithin:cholesterol acyltransferase reaction. *J Lipid Res* 9:155, 1968.

Gofman J, Glazier F, Tamplin A, et al: Lipoproteins, coronary heart disease and atherosclerosis. *Physiol Rev* 34:589, 1954.

Goldstein JL, Hazzard WR, Schrott HG, et al: Hyperlipidemia in coronary heart disease. I. Lipid levels in 500 survivors of myocardial infarction. *J Clin Invest* 52:1533–1543, 1973.

Goldstein JL, Kita T, Brown MS: Defective lipoprotein receptors and atherosclerosis: lessons from an animal counterpart of familial hypercholesterolemia. *N Engl J Med* 309:288, 1983.

Goldstein JL, Schrott HG, Hazzard WR, et al: Hyperlipidemia in coronary heart disease. II. Genetic analysis of lipid levels in 176 families and delineation of a new inherited disorder, combined hyperlipidemia. *J Clin Invest* 52:1544–1568, 1973.

Gotto AM, Gorry GA, Thompson JR, et al: Relationship between plasma lipid concentrations and coronary artery disease in 496 patients. *Circulation* 56:875–883, 1977.

Grundy SM: Pathogenesis of hyperlipoproteinemia. *J Lipid Res* 25:1611–1618, 1984.

Grundy SM, Vega GL: Causes of high blood cholesterol. *Circulation* (in press).

Grundy SM, Vega GL: Hypertriglyceridemia: causes and relation to coronary heart disease. *Seminars in Thrombosis and Hemostasis* 14:149–164, 1988.

Grundy SM, Chait A, Brunzell JD: Familial combined hyperlipidemia workshop. *Arteriosclerosis* 7:203–207, 1987.

Grundy SM, Mok HYI, Zech LA, et al: Transport of very low density lipoprotein-triglycerides in varying degrees of obesity and hypertriglyceridemia. *J Clin Invest* 63:1274–1283, 1979.

Grundy SM, Vega GL, Bilheimer DW: Causes and treatment of hypercholesterolemia, in Grundy SM (ed): *Bile Acids and Atherosclerosis*. Raven Press, New York, 1986, pp 13–40.

Grundy SM, Vega GL, Bilheimer DW: Kinetic mechanisms determining variability in low density lipoprotein levels and their rise with age. *Arteriosclerosis* 5:623–630, 1985.

Havel RJ: Familial dysbetalipoproteinemia: new aspects of pathogenesis and diagnosis. *Med Clin North Am* 66:441–454, 1982.

Havel RJ, Goldstein JL, Brown MS: Lipoproteins and lipid transport, in Bondy PK, Rosenberg LE (eds): *Metabolic Control and Disease*. WB Saunders, Philadelphia, 1980.

Hazzard WR, Goldstein JL, Schrott HG, et al: Hyperlipidemia in coronary heart disease. III. Lipoprotein phenotyping of 156 genetically defined survivors of myocardial infarction. *J Clin Invest* 52:1569–1577, 1973.

Howard BV: Lipoprotein metabolism in diabetes mellitus. *J Lipid Res* 28:613–628, 1987.

Hulley SB, Rosenman RH, Bawol RD, et al: Epidemiology as a guide to clinical decisions: the association between triglyceride and coronary heart disease. *N Engl J Med* 302:1383–1389, 1980.

Innerarity TL, Weisgraber KH, Arnold KS, et al: Familial defective apolipoprotein B-100: low density lipoproteins with abnormal receptor binding. *Proc Natl Acad Sci USA* 84:6919–6923, 1987.

Kesäniemi YA, Grundy SM: Dual defect in metabolism of very low density lipoprotein triglycerides in patients with type 5 hyperlipoproteinemia. *JAMA* 251:2542–2547, 1984.

Kesäniemi YA, Miettinen TA: Cholesterol absorption efficiency regulates plasma cholesterol level in the Finnish population. *Eur J Clin Invest* 17:391–395, 1987.

Kissebah AH, Alfarsi S, Evans DJ: Low density lipoprotein metabolism in familial combined hyperlipidemia: mechanism of the multiple lipoprotein phenotypic expression. *Arteriosclerosis* 4:614–624, 1984.

Laakso M, Voutilainen E, Sarlund H, et al: Serum lipids and lipoproteins in middle-aged non-insulin-dependent diabetics. *Atherosclerosis* 56:271–281, 1985.

Marsh JB: Lipoprotein metabolism in experimental nephrosis. *J Lipid Res* 25:1619–1623, 1984.

Miller NE: Why does plasma low density lipoprotein concentration in adults increase with age? *Lancet* 1:263–266, 1984.

National Center for Health Statistics; Fulwood R, Kalsbeck W, Rifkind B, et al: Total serum cholesterol levels of adults 20–74 years of age: United States, 1976–80. *Vital and Health Statistics*, Ser. II, No. 236.

DHHS Pub. No. (PHS) 86–1686. Public Health Service. US Government Printing Office, Washington, DC, May 1986.

Nikkila EA: Familial lipoprotein lipase deficiency and related disorders of chylomicron metabolism, in: Stanbury JS, Wyngaarden JB, Fredrickson DS, et al (eds): *The Metabolic Basis of Inherited Disease*, 5th ed. McGraw-Hill, New York, 1983, pp 622–642.

Nikkila EA, Kekki M: Plasma triglyceride transport kinetics in diabetes mellitus. *Metabolism* 22:1, 1973.

Nikkila EA, Kekki M: Polymorphism of plasma triglyceride kinetics in normal human adult subjects. *Acta Med Scand* 190:49, 1971.

Nikkila EA, Taskinen MR, Kekki M: Relation of plasma high density lipoprotein cholesterol to lipoprotein-lipase activity in adipose tissue and skeletal muscle of man. *Atherosclerosis* 29:497, 1987.

Richards EG, Grundy SM, Cooper K: Influence of plasma triglycerides on lipoprotein patterns in normal subjects and patients with coronary heart disease. *Am J Cardiol* 63:1214–1220, 1989.

Ruderman NB, Haudenschild C: Diabetes as an atherogenic factor. *Prog Cardiovasc Dis* 26:373–412, 1984.

Russell DW, Esser V, Hobbs HH: Molecular basis of familial hypercholesterolemia. *Arteriosclerosis* 9:8–12, 1989.

Sanfelippo M, Grundy SM, Henderson L: Transport of very low density lipoprotein triglyceride (VLDL-TG): comparison of hemodialysis and hemofiltration. *Kidney Int* 16:868, 1979.

Sniderman A, Wolfson C, Teng B, et al: Association of hyperapobetalipoproteinemia with endogenous hypertriglyceridemia and atherosclerosis. *Ann Intern Med* 97:833, 1982.

Utermann G, Langenbeck U, Beisiegel U, et al: Genetics of the apolipoprotein E system in man. *Am J Hum Genet* 32:339–347, 1980.

Utermann G, Vogelberg KH, Steinmetz A, et al: Polymorphism of apolipoprotein E. II. Genetics of hyperlipoproteinemia type III. *Clin Genet* 15:37–62, 1979.

Vega GL, Grundy SM: In vivo evidence for reduced binding of low density lipoproteins to receptors as a cause of primary moderate hypercholesterolemia. *J Clin Invest* 78:1410–1414, 1986.

Unit Three

Dietary Therapy of Hyperlipidemia

Ahrens EH, Hirsch J, Insull W, et al: The influence of dietary fats on serum-lipid levels in man. *Lancet* 1:943–953, 1957.

Anderson JT, Lawler A, Keys A: Weight gain from simple overeating. II. Serum lipids and blood volume. *J Clin Invest* 36:81–88, 1957.

Becker N, Illingworth DR, Alaupovic P, et al: Effects of saturated, monounsaturated, and omega-6 polyunsaturated fatty acids on plasma lipids, lipoproteins, and apoproteins in humans. *Am J Clin Nutr* 37:355–360, 1983.

Bennett M, Uauy R, Grundy SM: Dietary fatty acid effects on T cell mediated immunity in mice infected with mycoplasma pulmonis or carcinogens. *Am J Path* 126:103–113, 1987.

Bonanome A, Grundy SM: Effect of dietary stearic acid on plasma cholesterol and lipoprotein levels. *N Engl J Med* 318:1244–1248, 1988.

Caggiula AW, Christakis G, Farrand M, et al: The multiple risk factor intervention trial (MRFIT). IV. Intervention blood lipids. *Prev Med* 10:443–475, 1981.

Committee on Diet and Health, Food and Nutrition Board, Commission of Life Sciences, National Research Council. *Diet and Health: Implications for Reducing Chronic Disease Risk*. National Academy Press, Washington, DC, 1989.

Connor WE: Hypolipidemic effects of dietary omega-3 fatty acids in normal and hyperlipidemic humans: effectiveness and mechanisms, in Simopoulos AP, Kifer RR, Martin RE (eds): *Health Effects of Polyunsaturated Fatty Acids in Seafoods*. Academic Press, Orlando, Florida, 1986, pp 173–210.

Connor WE, Cerqueira MT, Connor RW, et al: The plasma lipids, lipoproteins, and diet of the Tarahumara Indians of Mexico. *Am J Clin Nutr* 31:1131–1142, 1978.

Crouse JR, Grundy SM: Effects of alcohol on plasma lipoproteins and cholesterol and triglyceride metabolism in man. *J Lipid Res* 25:486–496, 1984.

Egusa G, Beltz WF, Grundy SM, et al: Influence of obesity on the metabolism of apolipoprotein B in humans. *J Clin Invest* 76:596–603, 1985.

The Expert Panel. Report of the National Cholesterol Education Program Expert Panel on Detection, Evaluation and Treatment of High Blood Cholesterol in Adults. *Arch Intern Med* 148:36–69, 1988.

Fox JC, McGill HC Jr, Carey KD, et al: In vivo regulation of hepatic LDL receptor mRNA in the baboon: differential effects of saturated and unsaturated fat. *J Biol Chem* 262:7014–7020, 1987.

Garg A, Bonanome A, Grundy SM, et al: Comparison of a high-carbohydrate diet with a high-monounsaturated-fat diet in patients with non-insulin-dependent diabetes mellitus. *N Engl J Med* 319:829–864, 1988.

Garrison RJ, Wilson PW, Castelli WP, et al: Obesity and lipoprotein cholesterol in the Framingham offspring study. *Metabolism* 29:1053–1060, 1980.

Grundy SM: Comparison of monounsaturated fatty acids and carbohydrates for lowering plasma cholesterol. *N Engl J Med* 314:745–748, 1986.

Grundy SM: Effects of polyunsaturated fats on lipid metabolism in patients with hypertriglyceridemia. *J Clin Invest* 55:269–282, 1975.

Grundy SM, Ahrens EH Jr: The effects of unsaturated dietary fats on absorption, excretion, synthesis, and distribution of cholesterol in man. *J Clin Invest* 49:1135–1152, 1970.

Grundy SM, Vega GL: Plasma cholesterol responsiveness to saturated fatty acids. *Am J Clin Nutr* 47:822–824, 1988.

Grundy SM, et al: Rationale of the Diet Heart Statement of the American Heart Association. *Circulation* 65:839A–885A, 1982.

Grundy SM, Florentin L, Nix D, et al: Comparison of monounsaturated fatty acids and carbohydrates for reducing raised levels of plasma cholesterol in man. *Am J Clin Nutr* 47:965–969, 1988.

Grundy SM (ed), Gotto AM Jr, Pierman EL, et al: Recommendations for treatment of hyperlipidemia in adults. *Circulation* 69:1067A–1090A, 1984.

Harris WS, Connor WE, McMurry MP: The comparative reduction of the plasma lipids and lipoproteins by dietary polyunsaturated fats: salmon oil versus vegetable oils. *Metabolism* 32:179, 1983.

Hashim SA, Arteaga A, van Itallie TB: Effect of a saturated medium-chain triglyceride on serum-lipids in man. *Lancet* 1:1105–1108, 1960.

Hegsted DM, McGandy RB, Myers ML, et al: Quantitative effects of dietary fat on serum cholesterol in man. *Am J Clin Nutr* 17:281–295, 1965.

Jackson RL, Kashyap ML, Barnhart RL, et al: Influence of polyunsaturated and saturated fats on plasma lipids and lipoproteins in man. *Am J Clin Nutr* 39:589–597, 1984.

Kannel WB, Gordon T, Castelli WP: Obesity, lipids, and glucose intolerance: the Framingham study. *Am J Clin Nutr* 32:1238–1245, 1979.

Katan MB, Beynen AC, DeVries JH, et al: Existence of consistent hypo- and hyperresponders to dietary cholesterol in man. *Am J Epidemiol* 123:221–234, 1986.

Katan MB, Burns MAM, Glatz JFC, et al: Congruence of individual responsiveness to dietary cholesterol and to saturated fat in man. *J Lipid Res* 29:883–892, 1988.

Kesäniemi YA, Beltz WF, Grundy SM: Comparisons of metabolism of apolipoprotein B in normal subjects, obese patients, and patients with coronary heart disease. *J Clin Invest* 76:586–595, 1985.

Keys A: Coronary heart disease in seven countries. *Circulation* 41:I-1–I-211, 1970.

Keys A, Fidanza F: Serum cholesterol and relative body weight of coronary patients in different populations. *Circulation* 22:1091–1106, 1960.

Keys A, Anderson JT, Grande F: Serum cholesterol response to changes in the diet: IV. Particular saturated fatty acids in the diet. *Metabolism* 14:776–787, 1965.

Keys A, Anderson JT, Grande F: Prediction of serum-cholesterol responses of man to changes in fats in the diet. *Lancet* 2:959–966, 1957.

Keys A, Menotti A, Karvonen MJ, et al: The diet and 15-year death rate in the Seven Countries Study. *Am J Epidemiol* 124:903–915, 1986.

Kinsell LW, Michaels GD, Partridge JW, et al: Effect upon serum cholesterol and phospholipids of diets containing large amounts of vegetable fat. *J Clin Nutr* 1:244–251, 1953.

Knittle JL, Ahrens EH Jr: Carbohydrate metabolism in two forms of hyperglyceridemia. *J Clin Invest* 43:485–495, 1964.

Knuiman JT, West CE, Katan MB, et al: Total cholesterol and high density lipoprotein cholesterol levels in populations differing in fat and carbohydrate intake. *Arteriosclerosis* 7:612–619, 1987.

Mattson FH, Grundy SM: Comparison of effects of dietary saturated, monosaturated, and polyunsaturated fatty acids on plasma lipids and lipoproteins in man. *J Lipid Res* 26:194–202, 1985.

Melish J, Le N-A, Ginsberg H, et al: Dissociation of apoprotein B and triglyceride production in very-low density lipoproteins. *Am J Physiol* 239:E354–E362, 1980.

Mensink RP, Katan MB: Effect of a diet enriched with monounsaturated or polyunsaturated fatty acids on levels of low-density and high-density lipoprotein cholesterol in healthy men and women. *N Engl J Med* 321:436–441, 1989.

Mensink RP, Katan MB: Effect of monounsaturated fatty acids versus complex carbohydrates on high-density lipoproteins in healthy men and women. *Lancet* 1:122–125, 1987.

National Diet-Heart Study Research Group. The National Diet-Heart Study Final Report. *Circulation Monograph* 18:I-201, 1968.

Nestel PJ, Hirsh EZ: Mechanism of alcohol induced hypertriglyceridemia. *J Lab Clin Med* 66:357–365, 1965.

Nestel PJ, Connor WE, Reardon MF, et al: Suppression by diets rich in fish oil of very low density lipoprotein production in man. *J Clin Invest* 74:82, 1984.

Phillipson BE, Rothrock DW, Connor WE, et al: The reduction of plasma lipids, lipoproteins, and apoproteins in hypertriglyceridemic patients by dietary fish oils. *N Engl J Med* 312:1210, 1985.

Reiser R, Probstfield JL, Silvers A, et al: Plasma lipid and lipoprotein response of humans to beef fat, coconut oil and safflower oil. *Am J Clin Nutr* 42:190–197, 1985.

Shekelle RB, Shryrock AM, Paul O, et al: Diet, serum cholesterol, and death from coronary heart disease: the Western Electric study. *N Engl J Med* 304:65–70, 1981.

Shepherd J, Packard CJ, Grundy SM, et al: Effects of saturated and polyunsaturated fat diets on the chemical composition and metabolism of low density lipoproteins in man. *J Lipid Res* 21:91–99, 1980.

Shepherd J, Packard CJ, Patsch JR, et al: Effects of dietary polyunsaturated and saturated fat on the properties of high density lipoprotein and the metabolism of apolipoprotein A-I. *J Clin Invest* 60:1582–1592, 1978.

Spady DK, Dietschy JM: Dietary saturated triacylglycerols suppress hepatic low density lipoprotein receptors in the hamster. *Proc Natl Acad Sci USA* 82:4526–4530, 1985.

Stamler J: Overweight, hypertension, hypercholesterolemia and coronary heart disease, in Mananni M, Lewis B, Contaldo F (eds): *Medical Complications of Obesity*. Academic Press, London, 1979, pp 191–216.

Strong JP: Atherosclerosis in primates: introduction and overview. *Primates Med* 9:1–15, 1976.

Sturdevant RAL, Pearce ML, Dayton S: Increased prevalence of cholelithiasis in men ingesting a serum-cholesterol-lowering diet. *N Engl J Med* 288:24–27, 1973.

Vega GL, Groszek E, Wolf R, et al: Influence of polyunsaturated fats on composition of plasma lipoproteins and apolipoproteins. *J Lipid Res* 23:811–822, 1982.

Wolf R, Grundy SM: Influence of weight reduction on plasma lipoproteins in obese patients. *Arteriosclerosis* 3:160–169, 1983.

Unit Four

Drug Therapy of Hyperlipidemia

A co-operative trial in the primary prevention of ischaemic heart disease using clofibrate: report from the Committee of Principal Investigators. *Br Heart J* 40:1069–1118, 1978.

Baker SG, Jaffe BI, Meadelson D, et al: Treatment of homozygous familial hypercholesterolemia with probucol. *S Afr Med J* 62:7, 1982.

Bilheimer DW, Grundy SM, Brown MS, et al: Mevinolin and colestipol stimulate receptor-mediated clearance of low density lipoprotein from plasma in familial hypercholesterolemia heterozygotes. *Proc Natl Acad Sci USA* 80:4124–4128, 1983.

Blane GF, Bogaievsky Y, Bonnefous F: Fenofibrate: influence on circulating lipids and side-effects in medium and long-term clinical use, in Fears R, Prous JR (eds): *Pharmacological Control of Hyperlipidemia*. Science Publishers, SA, Barcelona, 1986, pp 187–216.

Blankenhorn DH, Nessim SA, Johnson RL, et al: Beneficial effects of combined colestipol-niacin therapy on coronary atherosclerosis and coronary venous bypass grafts. *JAMA* 257:3233–3240, 1987.

Brown WV, Dujovne CA, Farquhar JW, et al: Effects of fenofibrate on plasma lipids: double-blind, multicenter study in patients with type IIA or IIB hyperlipidemia. *Arteriosclerosis* 6:670–678, 1986.

Canner PL, Berge KG, Wenger NK, et al: Fifteen year mortality in Coronary Drug Project patients: long-term benefit with niacin. *J Am Coll Cardiol* 8:1245–1255, 1986.

Committee of Principal Investigators. WHO cooperative trial on primary prevention of ischemic heart disease with clofibrate to lower serum cholesterol: final mortality follow-up. *Lancet* 2:600, 1984.

Coronary Drug Project Research Group: Gallbladder disease as a side effect of drugs influencing lipid metabolism. *N Engl J Med* 296:1185–1190, 1977.

Coronary Drug Project Research Group. Clofibrate and niacin in coronary heart disease. *JAMA* 231:360–381, 1975.

DeGennes JL, Cairou F, Truffert J, et al: Long-term (over 5 years) treatment of primary hyperlipidemias by fenofibrate alone or with cholestyramine, in Carlson LA, Olsson AG (eds): *Treatment of Hyperlipoproteinemia*. Raven Press, New York, 1984, p 175.

Dujoune CA, Krehbiel P, Decoursey S, et al: Probucol with colestipol in the treatment of hypercholesterolemia. *Ann Intern Med* 100:477, 1984.

East C, Alivizatos PA, Grundy SM, et al: Rhabdomyolysis in patients receiving lovastatin after cardiac transplantation. *N Engl J Med* 318:47–48, 1988.

Eisenberg S, Gavish D, Oschry Y, et al: Abnormalities in very low-, low- and high-density lipoproteins in hypertriglyceridemia: reversal toward normal with bezafibrate treatment. *J Clin Invest* 74:470–482, 1984.

Frick MH, Elo O, Haapa K, et al: Helsinki Heart Study: primary-prevention trial with gemfibrozil in middle-aged men with dyslipidemia: safety of treatment, changes in risk factors, and incidence of coronary heart disease. *N Engl J Med* 317:1237–1245, 1987.

Garg A, Grundy SM: Lovastatin for lowering cholesterol levels in noninsulin-dependent diabetes mellitus. *N Engl J Med* 318:81–86, 1988.

Gnasso A, Lehner B, Haberbosch W, et al: Effect of gemfibrozil on lipids, apoproteins, and postheparin lipolytic activities in normolipidemic subjects. *Metabolism* 35:387–393, 1986.

Grundy SM: HMG-CoA reductase inhibitors for treatment of hypercholesterolemia. *N Engl J Med* 319:24–33, 1988.

Grundy SM: Treatment of hypercholesterolemia by interference with bile acid metabolism. *Arch Intern Med* 130:638–648, 1972.

Grundy SM, Mok HYI: Colestipol, clofibrate, and phytosterols in combined therapy of hyperlipidemia. *J Lab Clin Med* 89:354–366, 1977.

Grundy SM, Vega GL: Fibric acids: effects on lipids and lipoprotein metabolism. *Am J Med* 83(suppl 5B):9–20, 1987.

Grundy SM, Vega GL: Influence of mevinolin on metabolism of low-denisty lipoproteins in primary moderate hypercholesterolemia. *J Lipid Res* 26:1464–1475, 1985.

Grundy SM, Ahren EGJ, Salen G, et al: Mechanism of action of clofibrate on cholesterol metabolism in patients with hyperlipidemia. *J Lipid Res* 13:531–551, 1972.

Grundy SM, Goodman DEW, Rifkind BM, et al: The place of HDL in cholesterol management: a perspective from the National Cholesterol Education Program. *Arch Intern Med* 149:505–510, 1989.

Grundy SM, Mok HYI, Zech L, et al: Influence of nicotinic acid on metabolism of cholesterol and triglycerides in man. *J Lipid Res* 22:24–36, 1981.

Grundy SM, Vega GI, Bilheimer DW: Influence of combined therapy with mevinolin and interruption of bile-acid reabsorption on low density lipoproteins in heterozygous familial hypercholesterolemia. *Ann Intern Med* 103:339–343, 1985.

Havel RJ, Hunninghake DB, Illingworth DR, et al: Lovastatin (mevinolin) in the treatment of heterozygous familial hypercholesterolemia: a multicenter study. *Ann Intern Med* 107:609–615, 1987.

Hunninghake DB: Drug interactions involving hypolipidemic drugs, in Petrie JC (ed): *Cardiovascular and Respiratory Disease Therapy*. Elsevier/North Holland, New York, 1980, p 79.

Hunninghake DB, Probstfield JL: Drug treatment of hyperlipoproteinemia, in *Hyperlipidemia—Diagnosis and Therapy*. Grune and Stratton, New York, 1977, p 327.

Hunninghake DB: Resin therapy: adverse effects and their management, in Fears R, Prous JR (eds): *Pharmacological Control of Hyperlipidemia*. Science Publishers, SA, Barcelona, 1986, pp 67–89.

Illingworth DR: Mevinolin plus colestipol in therapy for severe heterozygous familial hypercholesterolemia. *Ann Intern Med* 101:598–604, 1984.

Illingworth DR, Sexton GJ: Hypocholesterolemic effects of mevinolin in patients with heterozygous familial hypercholesterolemia. *J Clin Invest* 74:1972–1978, 1984.

Kane JP, Malloy MJ: Treatment of hypercholesterolemia. *Med Clin North Am* 66:537–550, 1982.

Kane JP, Malloy MJ, Tun P, et al: Normalization of low-density-lipoprotein levels in heterozygous familial hypercholesterolemia with a combined drug regimen. *N Engl J Med* 304:251–258, 1981.

Kesäniemi YA, Grundy SM: Influence of probucol on cholesterol and lipoprotein metabolism in man. *J Lipid Res* 25:780–790, 1984.

Kesäniemi YA, Beltz WF, Grundy SM: Comparisons of clofibrate and caloric restriction on transport of very low density lipoprotein triglycerides. *Arteriosclerosis* 5:153–161, 1985.

Kita T, Nagano Y, Yokode M, et al: Probucol prevents the progression of atherosclerosis in Watanabe heritable hyperlipidemic rabbit, an animal model for familial hypercholesterolemia. *Proc Natl Acad Sci USA* 84:5928–5931, 1987.

Knapp RH, Ginsberg J, Albers JJ, et al: Contrasting effects of unmodified and time-release forms of niacin on lipoproteins in hyperlipidemic subjects: clues to mechanism of action of niacin. *Metabolism* 34:642, 1985.

Levy RI, Brensike JF, Epstein SE, et al: The influence of changes in lipid values induced by cholestyramine and diet on progression of coronary artery disease: results of the NHLBI Type II Coronary Intervention Study. *Circulation* 69:325–337, 1984.

Lipid Research Clinics Program. The Lipid Research Clinics Coronary Primary Prevention Trial results. I. Reduction in incidence of coronary heart disease. *JAMA* 251:351–364, 1984.

Lipid Research Clinics Program. The Lipid Research Clinics Coronary Primary Prevention Trial results. II. The relationship of reduction in incidence of coronary heart disease to cholesterol lowering. *JAMA* 251:365–374, 1984.

Lovastatin Study Group II. Therapeutic response to lovastatin (mevinolin) in nonfamilial hypercholesterolemia: a multicenter study. *JAMA* 256:2829–2834, 1986.

Manninen V, Elo MO, Frick MH, et al: Lipid alterations and decline in the incidence of coronary heart disease in the Helsinki Heart Study. *JAMA* 260:641–651, 1988.

Mol MJTM, Erkelens DW, Gevers Leuven JA, et al: Effects of synovinolin (MK-733) on plasma lipids in familial hypercholesterolemia. *Lancet* 2:936–939, 1986.

Norman DJ, Illingworth DR, Munson J, et al: Myolysis and acute renal failure in a heart-transplant recipient receiving lovastatin. *N Engl J Med* 318:46–47, 1988.

Olsson AG, Walldius G, Wahlberg G: Pharmacological control of hyperlipidemia: nicotinic acid and its analogues—mechanisms of action, effects and clinical usage, in Fears R, Prous JR (eds): *Pharmacological Control of Hyperlipidemia*. Science Publishers, SA, Barcelona, 1986, pp 217–230.

Packard CJ, Shepherd J: The hepatobiliary axis and lipoprotein metabolism: effects of bile acid sequestrants and ilial bypass surgery. *J Lipid Res* 23:1081, 1982.

Saku K, Gartside PS, Hynd BA, et al: Mechanism of action of gemfibrozil on lipoprotein metabolism. *J Clin Invest* 75:1702–1712, 1985.

Shepherd J, Packard CJ: An overview of the effects of p-chlorophenoxyisobutyric acid derivatives on lipoprotein metabolism, in Fears R, Prous JR (eds): *Pharmacological Control of Hyperlipidaemia*. Science Publishers, SA, Barcelona, Spain, 1986, pp 135–144.

Stewart JM, Packard CJ, Lorimer AR, et al: Effects of bezafibrate on receptor-mediated and receptor-independent low density lipoprotein catabolism in type II hyperlipoproteinemic subjects. *Atherosclerosis* 44:355–365, 1982.

Taylor KG, Holdsworth G, Dalton DJ: Clofibrate increases lipoprotein lipase activity in adipose tissue of hypertriglyceridaemic patients. *Lancet* II:1106, 1977.

Tobert JA, Bell GD, Birtwell J, et al: Cholesterol-lowering effect of mevinolin, an inhibitor of 3-hydroxy-3-methylglutaryl coenzyme A reductase, in healthy volunteers. *J Clin Invest* 69:913–919, 1982.

Uauy R, Vega GL, Grundy SM, et al: Lovastatin therapy in receptor-negative homozygous familial hypercholesterolemia: lack of effect on low density lipoprotein concentrations or turnover. *J Pediatr* (in press).

Vega GL, Grundy SM: Comparison of lovastatin and gemfibrozil in normolipidemic patients with hypoalphalipoproteinemia. *JAMA* 262:3148–3153, 1989.

Vega GL, Grundy SM: Lovastatin therapy in nephrotic hyperlipidemia: effects on lipoprotein metabolism. *Kidney Int* 33:1160–1168, 1988.

Vega GL, Grundy SM, Treatment of primary moderate hypercholesterolemia with lovastatin (mevinolin) and colestipol. *JAMA* 257:33–38, 1987.

Vega GL, East C, Grundy SM: Lovastatin therapy in familial dysbetalipoproteinemia: effects on kinetics of apolipoprotein B. *Atherosclerosis* 70:131–143, 1988.

Yamamoto A, Matsuzaw Y, Kishino B, et al: Effects of probucol on homozygous cases of familial hypercholesterolemia. *Atherosclerosis* 48:157, 1983.

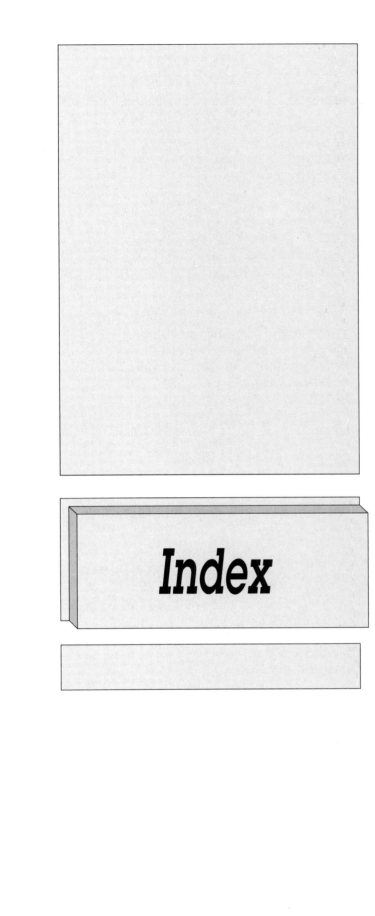

Index

Index

Note:

The numbers set in **boldface** type refer to figure numbers.